Dis-Solving Conflict from Within

Dis-Solving Conflict from Within

AN INNER PATH FOR CONFLICT TRANSFORMATION

Henry Yampolsky

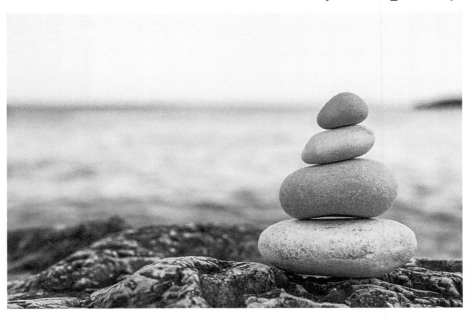

GLOBAL
COLLECTIVE
PUBLISHERS

Published by Global Collective Publishers, LLC
16 North Bryn Mawr Avenue, #1355
Bryn Mawr, Pennsylvania 19010, U.S.A.
www.globalcollectivepublishers.com

Hardback ISBN: 978-1-7344019-4-3
eBook ISBN: 978-1-7344019-5-0

To Juliya and
To Anand, the two teachers who have influenced me the most

TABLE OF CONTENTS

FOREWORD¹

At the time of profound divisions and incessant conflicts, many conflict resolution books offer suggestions for making our divisions less visible and conflicts more tolerable. My friend and colleague, Henry Yampolsky takes a different aim in this fresh and needed work. He challenges us to transform our conflict interactions by looking within each and every one of us.

This path involves commitment to a regular practice of tuning inward, observation without evaluation, expansion and exploration. Henry emphasizes the importance of tuning inward by presenting a simple but powerful mindfulness-based process for developing self-awareness in conflict. It is self-awareness and contentment with what is which enables us to *respond* to conflict with "strength, clarity, and ease." And indeed, it is this long-term awareness that serves as a preventative measure for conflict. That's not to say that conflict won't ever happen, but using the "Dis-Solving Conflict from Within" method can certainly empower one to move from a reaction to a response in conflict and serve to prevent future conflicts.

In my experience, vulnerability, awareness, and humility—are signs of an expert mediator. Henry exhibits all these qualities in his book. Moreover, I have learned that a mediator's job is more than helping parties reach a resolution; it's about connecting with people's emotions—and it is apparent from reading *Dis-Solving Conflict from Within* that Henry values this, as he places it at the center of his method. He has a genuine desire for peace, and he works towards this goal by helping one to develop inner peace through introspection and self-reflection.

Henry is also a keen student of Eastern teachings and traditions, sharing them in a way which is respectful to their origin, ever practical but never preachy or esoteric. He is also an engaging storyteller who sprinkles pieces of his narrative which involved immigration to the U.S. from Ukraine; frustration with being a trial lawyer; many journeys to India to study Yoga and meditation; learning to ride motorcycles as a way to find passion in life, and even riding one across the Himalayas. Henry's determination to find inner peace, his humility, and humanity truly lead by example.

Henry's narrative, his examples, and prescriptions invite us to conclude that not only everything we do matters, no matter how big or how small, but that the source of our actions is of critical importance. Ultimately this book provides us with the ability to change the way in which we approach life from the lofts of our "tiny skull-sized kingdoms."[2] Rather than approach life as if we are the center of the universe, and life revolves around us, Henry's inward journey—both his own and the one he invites readers on, empowers one to connect with the innate humanity and universal needs of our conflict partners, whether they are across the table, across cultures, or on different sides of a political, social or cultural divide from us. This stems from a profound insight that truly puts the whole book into perspective—we and our conflict partners are something much more than our ideas, beliefs, experiences, roles, prejudices or preferences. In other words, we cannot reduce a person's identity to a stereotype, prejudice, or opinion they hold which we may not agree with. With this realization we can no longer see conflict in simplistic and divisive us-versus-them terms. This is what transforms conflict and fundamentally alters our conflict interactions. This view is crucial because, while we all hail from different cultures and walks of life, we are ultimately part of one global community, one interconnected universe. We already have all the tools to eliminate division and foster this unified community. These tools are within us. If you are interested in exploring and utilizing these tools, you will enjoy your journey to dis-solving conflict from within.

INTRODUCTION

Recently, a friend invited me to a dinner party. The first part of her invitation read as follows:

Aren't you tired of arguing?
Come share good food and some cheer!
The party's theme this year is tolerance and civility!

I swallowed hard as I read the above phrase. It wasn't just the odd rhyming. I knew my friend's intentions were pure and reflected the sentiments I hear so often now—"we are exhausted from fighting!" "can't we just get along?!" "I'm dreading Thanksgiving this year!" "I feel I can no longer talk without shouting to the people I care deeply about." However, it was the words "tolerance" and "civility" that were the most triggering for me. If I said to you, my wife and I tolerate each other, would you be happy for me? How about if I shared that we are civil with each other? I'd like to have a lot more color, juice, spice, and sparkle in my marriage and when gathering with friends than merely being tolerant or civil.

The focus on tolerance and civility reflects a fundamental belief that conflict is some force outside of us we must avoid or escape or, at a minimum, manage with great care. My intention with this book is to challenge this belief. I don't see conflict as some force outside of us, happening *to* us. Rather, I see conflict as a reflection of *how we are* and of *what is happening within us.* What is happening within us is profound confusion between what is *us* and what is *ours*. We identify with all sorts of accumulations such as our beliefs, judgements, preferences, prejudices, and philosophies. As a result, any challenge to these beliefs, judgements, preferences, prejudices, and philosophies feels like a direct threat and a challenge to us. We compulsively react to these perceived threats and challenges by trying to escape, avoid, or dominate them and end up letting each and every thing which triggers us control our lives. Consequently, we are then fearful, anxious, disengaged, entangled, and deeply steeped in the idea of separation—the illusion that each of us is a distinct island with no connection with or responsibility for each other—separate from the very life that we are and the world we are an integral part of. This in turn creates the world steeped in cruelty, injustice, and lack, dominated by a simplistic "us" vs. "them" paradigm.

The ultimate invitation of this book is to turn inward. I suggest that turning inward, rather than focusing outside of us, is what enables us to respond to conflict with strength, clarity, and ease, instead of reacting to it with fear, avoidance, or aggression. Responding to conflict and life's other challenges means moving from a compulsive action to a conscious one. Acting consciously from an undisturbed state is what transforms our conflict interactions from destructive experiences we dread and fear to constructive opportunities for transformative growth, for meaningful connections, and for insightful and interesting dialogues.

I see turning inward in conflict not merely as an abstract idea but as an intentional life path. My hope is that this book provides as much direction as possible towards this path. Thus, the first two parts of the book will explore what I see as the more holistic way of seeing conflict and then will introduce the Dis-Solving Conflict from Within™ process. Dis-Solving Conflict from Within™ process is a simple four-step self-inquiry tool for going inward in conflict. In a very subtle way, it creates some space between the critical components of conflict and us. Creating, exploring, and deepening this space begins the process of dis-solving our enduring inner conflict—the consistently persistent confusion between what is *ours* and what is *us*. As this confusion dis-solves, we start seeing people and situations as they are and develop the capacity to take appropriate, decisive action from a clear and undisturbed state. This fundamentally changes how we are and thus radically transforms our conflict interactions.

In Part Three of this book, we zoom out and examine the four-part framework for transforming conflict. This framework consists of principles of tuning inward, observation without evaluation, expansion, and exploration as well as of the practices which integrate these principles into our day-to-day lives and interactions. Part Four of this book introduces three specific tools: Compassionate Communications, Restorative Dialogues, and Mediation. These tools further integrate the conflict transformation framework and offer concrete ways for constructively engaging in and responding to conflict. While I introduce these tools, the chapters which describe them are not designed to be "how to" manuals on using these tools. In the Resources Section I link to training, books, and other materials which explore each of these tools in greater detail. The examples I use in this book are based on many complex conflicts I've worked with, though to protect the privacy of individuals who entrusted their conflicts to me, where possible, names and identifying details have been changed. Also, nothing in this book is intended to or designed for treating any physical or mental condition. Those recovering from past trauma and/or those with symptoms of PTSD, severe depression and other mental health conditions should utilize the Dis-Solving Conflict from Within™ Process only under strict supervision by a licensed mental health professional.

My personal path for turning inward took me from West to East. Trained as a lawyer in America, I became deeply dissatisfied with the Western approach to conflict and felt drained by the American, adversarial approach to the practice of law. A series of transformative events, which I describe in this book, took me to India where I became exposed to profound, universal, timeless, and enduring teachings which completely transformed my worldview and placed me on the path within. These teachings, as presented by two incredible beings, my teacher Anand Mehrotra and Sadhguru Jaggi Vasudev, are at the very core of this book. Though my path is influenced by the East, this book neither advocates for nor requires any particular set of beliefs.

The more steps inward I took, the more I realized how living from within can not only transform ourselves or our interpersonal conflicts, but can also influence complex and enduring global issues we face as humans. Ultimately, the world we live in, with all of its problems, is not separate from how we are. Thus, by changing ourselves and by transforming our conflict interactions we can radically transform the world, ensuring that future generations will not only survive, but will have an opportunity to thrive on a planet steeped in compassion, unity, collaboration, and peace.

Also, the more inward steps I take, the more I realize how little I know about everything. Although this book represents my life's work, my insight and understanding are ever evolving. Any wisdom contained in the following pages flowed through me and thus is not "mine." However, all mistakes, misquotes, misinterpretations, misunderstandings, and opinions expressed are mine alone. I have ways to go in fully living all the lessons in this book. Yet, I know with every fiber of my being that we as people, as humanity, could do a lot better than tolerance and civility. The only way forward is in. The pages that follow offer the path within.

Part One

UNDERSTANDING CONFLICT

1

OF MICE AND US

Animal behaviorist John Calhoun began one of the most famous experiments in psychology by dropping four pairs of mice into a 9 by 4.5-foot metal pan. Each side of the pan had four groups of four vertical, wire mesh "tunnels." The "tunnels" gave access to nesting boxes, food hoppers, and water dispensers. There was no shortage of food, water, or nesting material. There were no predators. Calhoun's metal pen became known as "mice utopia."

Initially, the rodent population in the mice utopia experienced rapid growth, doubling every 55 days. At approximately the 300-day mark, when the population in the pen passed 600 mice, Calhoun observed increased conflict, anti-social, and destructive behavior among mice. In the study he first published in 1962, Calhoun described this phenomenon as follows:

Many [female mice] were unable to carry pregnancy to full term or to survive delivery of their litters if they did. An even greater number, after successfully giving birth, fell short in their maternal functions. Among the males the behavior disturbances ranged from sexual deviation to cannibalism and from frenetic overactivity to a pathological withdrawal from which individuals would emerge to eat, drink and move about only when other members of the community were asleep. The social organization of the animals showed equal disruption. ...[3]

The mice population peaked at 2,200 before beginning to decline. The social breakdown, marked by increased withdrawal by individual mice from any communal interactions, persisted as mice engaged only in the tasks essential to their health. They ate, drank, slept, and groomed themselves, but showed no interest in breeding or in other social interactions. By day 600 the mice utopia was moving towards extinction. Soon, mice utopia and its inhabitants were no more.[4] John Calhoun and many others drew parallels between "mice utopia" and the world we inhabit. We'll talk a bit later about Calhoun's conclusions, but first let's explore the striking similarities between mice and us.

As the world population has passed 7 billion, the technological and scientific advances over the past hundred years have created lives for us that our ancestors could not even imagine living. To satisfy our basic needs—food, water, procreation—we only need to swipe right, left, up, or down on our phone. From the palm of our hand, we can access the greatest works of literature and art, and the deepest wisdom from every tradition. We could converse in full, HD-Video with someone halfway around the world and call someone we've never met most vile names on Twitter or Facebook. We could accomplish all this and a lot more without ever leaving our couch.

Should we be inclined to get up, we likely live in a temperature-controlled home with easy access to modern conveniences and endless entertainment options. Our cars are also temperature and computer-controlled boxes that can whisk us away, with increasingly little effort and involvement from us. Should we be inclined to venture further, a pressurized metal tube could fly us and our luggage in relative comfort nearly anywhere in the world. In fact, in twenty-four hours or less we could travel between just about any two points on the planet.

It is undeniable that our lives are more convenient than anyone could have imagined possible one hundred or even fifty years ago. Like in John Calhoun's mice paradise, in many places around the world, and at least for now, there is ample food and water. Likewise, aside from fellow humans, who do the cruelest of things to each other, no predators present a threat to us.

Yet, "utopia" or "paradise" would hardly be the words that describe the experience of most humans. In fact, over the past decades, if there were words that could capture the human experience on this planet, these words would be conflict, division, stress, and ever-increasing polarization.

Conflict seems to be an especially poignant description of the years 2020 and 2021. As I write these words, hundreds of millions of people around the world have contracted the coronavirus COVID-19.[5] Over five million people have died to date due to this deadly pathogen. Over 748,000 people have died in the United States; 459,000 in India; and 608,000 in Brazil.[6] The COVID-19 pandemic has highlighted the long-simmering conflict between "haves" and "have nots" around the world. It is the "have nots" that bore the brunt of the direct and indirect impacts of the COVID-19 pandemic.[7] The COVID-19 pandemic itself is evidence of a long-standing and escalating conflict between humans and the environment. Human activity is responsible for the loss of up to 150 species of plants and animals every day.[8] The Global Assessment Report on Biodiversity and Ecosystem Services estimated in 2019 that nearly 1 million species of animals and plants will face extinction in the next decade due to human activity.[9] With these devastating losses, it is of little surprise that animal viruses, like COVID-19, have fewer and fewer animal hosts, and thus are migrating to humans.[10]

There also have not been any shortages in political and social upheaval around the world. The bitter 2016 American presidential contest and the subsequent presidency of Donald J. Trump exposed deep seated divisions, grievances, inequities, and resentments among various slices of American society. The challenges of coping with the continuous impacts of the pandemic; the recent murders of unarmed, Black Americans in the prime of their lives—William Green, Jaquyn O'Neill Light, Lionell Morris, Ahmaud Arbery, Manuel Ellis, Barry Gedeus, Breonna Taylor, Daniel Prude, Steven Taylor, Cornelius Fredericks, Maurice Gordon, George Floyd, Dion Johnson, Tony McDade, Calvin Horton, Jr., James Scurlock, David McAtee, Jamel Floyd, Kamal Flowers, Robert Forbes, Priscila Slater, Rayshard Brooks, Maurice Abisdid-Wagner, Julian Lewis, Anthony McClain, Damian Daniels, and Dijon Kizzee; the January 6th, 2021 storming of the U.S. Capitol; continued economic woes; and the ever-present political gridlock in Washington all served to amplify these divisions, grievances, inequities, injustices, and resentments among Americans.

America is hardly alone in seeing an increase in political and social upheaval. As I write these words Russia is waging an all-out war against my home country of Ukraine. China has jailed and killed thousands of Muslim Uighurs and has reasserted its power and cultural, political, and military dominance over Tibet.[11] Myanmar has underwent a military coup.[12] Haiti is living through a devastating upheaval following the July 2021 assassination of President Jovenel Moïse. After twenty years of American involvement in Afghanistan, thousands of lives lost, and billions of dollars spent, Taliban is once again fully controlling the country.

Inner turmoil and conflict are also tormenting millions of people around the world. Between 1990 and 2017, an estimated 264 million people in the world suffered from depression.[13] This number is expected to grow exponentially during and after the COVID-19 crisis.[14] Just in the U.S. there are on average 132 suicides per day, with suicide now being the 10th leading cause of death in America.[15] In India, over 200,000 people took their lives in 2016.[16] In China, suicide is the fifth leading cause of death and accounts for over one-quarter of suicides worldwide.[17] Suicide rates are comparably high in Russia, South Korea, Japan, Belgium, Kazakhstan, and Belarus.[18]

The United States is also in the midst of the worst drug addiction epidemic in its history. Prescriptions for and deaths from opioids both quadrupled between 1995 and 2010. By 2015, an estimated 92 million individuals in the United States were prescribed an opioid and there were more than 33000 deaths from an opioid-involved overdose.[19] 2018 data shows that every day, 128 people in the United States die after overdosing on opioids.[20] Curiously, unlike PSP and other drugs of the 1960s, which people took for greater clarity, opioids are dulling drugs—drugs designed to dull both physical and emotional pain. In fact, according to the 2015 Princeton University study there has been a marked increase in the "deaths of despair"—death by drugs, alcohol, and suicide especially among white, middle-aged males with a high school education or less.[21]

The above statistics only provide a small glimpse of the multitude of conflicts we are experiencing. Of course, these do not include many "day-to-day" conflicts and microaggressions that occur at work; with intimate partners; with acquaintances or friends; or are a result of implicit and systemic biases. And we don't need any statistics to tell us how polarized and divided we are as people and how deeply ingrained and thus threatened many of our identities, beliefs, judgments, and preferences have become.

So, are we just like mice in John Calhoun's experiment, living in a utopia while obliviously moving towards our own extinction? Maybe, or maybe not.

Of course, it is easy to dismiss mice as primitive creatures that are nothing like us. Such a quick dismissal would be a mistake. On the most basic level, just like mice and other creatures, we are born and then we spend our lives satisfying our basic needs—for food, for shelter, and for occasional pleasure. Yes, we have language, logic, deep thoughts, and complex emotions! So do mice and other mammals.[22] While animal language, logic, thought, and emotions might not have the same variety and depth as ours, there is no denying that animals use these faculties just as we do.[23] In fact, we humans share about 97.5% of our working DNA with mice.[24]

However, there is one critical difference between mice and us. Whereas animals are programmed to *react* to stimuli in a particular way—through fear, avoidance, or aggression, we have an innate ability to *respond*. Our ability to respond, or *response-ability*, means that in any situation we can choose how to be; that regardless of what is happening for us, we can choose our inner experience. Austrian psychologist and neurologist Viktor Frankl, who witnessed his family perish in the Holocaust and himself survived a Nazi concentration camp, described response-ability in his book *Man's Search for Meaning* as follows:

> Everything can be taken from a man but one thing: the last of human freedoms—to choose one's attitude in any given set of circumstances, to choose one's own way.

Spiritual teacher and best-selling author, Wayne Dyer agreed, noting that: "[y]ou cannot always control what goes on outside. But you can always control what goes on inside." There is a widely circulated story about Lao Tzu, the ancient mystic and philosopher who founded Taoism. Lao Tzu was widely persecuted and by all accounts had a very difficult life. As Lao Tzu was nearing the end of his life his students gathered around him soaking in their beloved Master's last words of wisdom. One student asked: "Master, you've had many struggles in your life, yet you are one of the happiest people we all know. What is the secret to your happiness?" Lao Tzu responded: "Every day of my life I woke up and asked myself one simple question—shall I be joyous today or shall I be miserable? So far, everyday I've chosen to be joyous."

At the very core of our ability to respond lies the most profound choice—do we focus within or outside of us? Focus outside of us means that outside factors determine *how* we are in any particular situation. Thus, if the weather or our neighbor are nice, then we are nice, if the sky or our partner's mood turns cloudy, dreariness overcomes us. Focus outside of us reduces us to a set of compulsive reactions. Like software, these same reactions get activated every time something or someone triggers us. And since there is always someone or something out there to trigger us, that someone or something holds a remote control to us.

Focus outside of us has a much greater impact than merely determining our mood at a particular point in time. I suggest that focus outside of us is largely responsible for the majority of our world's problems and calamities, a few of which I noted above. Because focus outside of us perpetuates three very harmful, deeply held, and very influential beliefs. These beliefs are: that we have a set, limited identity, defined by our accumulations, especially the accumulations of the body and the mind; that each of us is, in essence, an island—separate, special, distinct, and disconnected from everything and everyone else; and that that our life is both infinite and transitory, meaning that we have unlimited time and are, anyway, just passing through on our way to some other "better" place.

World renown Indian mystic and *New York Times* best-selling author Sadhguru Jaggi Vasudev speaks often in his many wisdom talks (widely available on YouTube and other social media platforms) on the nature of identity. Sadhguru points out that our body is an accumulation of genetic information and bio-memories we've gathered through generations and of food we've gathered in this lifetime. Likewise, Sadghuru teaches, our mind is an accumulation of ideas, judgements, prejudices, conditioning, beliefs, and philosophies we've gathered. Thus, while both are *ours*, neither is *us*. Of course, the same is true of our social and familial roles, education, careers, status, our physical possessions, and even political identities and religious beliefs—all are accumulations. If we saw them as merely accumulations, and not as *us*, would we fight all these wars and commit senseless and most cruel acts of violence over them? In something as simple and life-sustaining as our breath, we are completely dependent on Earth's atmosphere having just the right mixture of oxygen for us. In fact, whether we like somebody or not, we inhale what they exhale and they inhale what we exhale. The cycles of a distant moon govern the cycles of a woman's body, and thus are responsible for our very life. Every grain of food we consume originated somewhere else. If pesky insects were to disappear from this planet, so would human life. If the sun changed its temperature by just a few degrees or Earth slightly shifted its tilt, all of us would be gone. A tiny virus brings all kinds of havoc into our lives. These small observations about the nature of our existence are evidence of a now well-established scientific fact—we are part of an infinitely interconnected and interdependent universe.

As noted by philosopher of science Ervin Laszlo and cosmologist Jude Currivan in their book, *CosMos: A Co-creator's Guide to the Whole World*,

> We are beginning to see the entire universe as a holographically interlinked network of energy and information, organically whole and self-referential at all scales of its existence. We, and all things in the universe, are non-locally connected with each other and with all other things in ways that are unfettered by the hitherto known limitations of space and time.

If instead of seeing ourselves as separate, distinct, special, and unique islands, we start experiencing ourselves as an integral part of a greater whole, does it not fundamentally change the way we interact with the environment and with each other? Biologist Elisabet Sahtouris in her article, "Biology of Globalization", responded:

> We must see ourselves in community with all other people at local, national and global levels. While this may seem superficially easy, it is actually not. Western culture, now globally dominant, has systematically trained us to think and act as though we are separate individuals, often in competition with each other for scarce resources of one sort or another, primarily money, which has become the perceived means to all we want and need in life.[25]

Finally, Albert Einstein famously said:

> A human being is a part of the whole called by us universe, a part limited in time and space. He experiences himself, his thoughts and feelings as something separated from the rest, a kind of optical delusion of his consciousness. This delusion is a kind of prison for us, restricting us to our personal desires and to affection for a few persons nearest to us. Our task must be to free ourselves from this prison by widening our circle of compassion to embrace all living creatures and the whole of nature in its beauty.

And, we are not so special! In relation to our Galaxy (and there are many others beyond ours), Planet Earth is a tiny dot. New York City or Mumbai are micro-dots on this tiny dot. We are micro-specks of dust on these micro-dots. Our life-span of 70-80 years is but a blink of an eye, over before it begins. Yet, within this reality we see ourselves as so special, big, and important and act as though our lives will never end. In fact, many of us consume for multiple lifetimes. To paraphrase Dalai Lama, we live as though we are never going to die and then die never having truly lived.

There is an alternative to this rat race of ours; to the "mice utopia" on the way to extinction and oblivion. The alternative is to turn within. That is the fundamental invitation of this book. Because regardless of whether we are dealing with a problem of global proportions such as COVID-19 or with our own untamed mind, which is very local to us, the sources of both problems are within us. As noted by the New York Times best-selling author, Michael A. Singer in his book, *Untethered Soul: The Journey Beyond Yourself,*

> The only permanent solution to your problems is to go inside and let go of the part of you that seems to have so many problems with reality. Once you do that, you'll be clear enough to deal with what's left.

The Dalai Lama often teaches that "world peace must develop from inner peace" with inner peace being "the manifestation of human compassion." Going within means that we take absolute, unconditional, and radical responsibility for our inner experience, *regardless of what is happening in the world outside of us.* Ironically, turning inward is the opposite of self-absorption. It actually is the most direct pathway to expanding our very idea of who we are. It is a way to experience ourselves as something greater than all of our many accumulations, as something inseparable from the vast world outside of us. Turning inward is a way of being more, not less, inclusive of all dimensions and expressions of life. As indirect as this path seems, it is the quickest and the most effective way to radically transform our inner, interpersonal, and global conflicts—because it begins and ends with transforming *us.*

So, while Dis-Solving Conflict from Within is a simple four-step process for turning inward in conflict, it must be viewed in the greater context of *living from within.* In this context Dis-Solving Conflict from Within is but one small, introductory step for turning inward. Thus, while this book will devote a considerable amount of space to introducing and teaching this process, ultimately it is not about Dis-Solving Conflict from Within as a process but about dis-solving conflict from within—turning inward when life challenges us—as a way of life.

Turning inward is not an escape from life's challenges, rather it is a complete embrace of our inner experiences of these challenges. Thus, as we will explore in later chapters, Dis-Solving Conflict from Within, both as a process and as an approach to life, is not a way to feel better. Rather, it is a way to get better at feeling all that is arising within us—experiences that are pleasant, and especially those that are not. Training ourselves to *unconditionally* (without trying to fix, change, or escape) feel all that is arising within us is key to not letting our experiences define us. In other words, it is the key to responding to life.

Coming back to John Calhoun's mice experiment for a moment. The conclusion that John Calhoun and many others drew from the "mice utopia" was the danger of overpopulation. While the mice population peaked at 2200, the paradise could actually easily sustain more than 3,000 mice. I think there is more than numbers at play here. When stressed and triggered, mice turned to compulsive reactions of fear, avoidance, and aggression. This brought the beginning of the end for the mice. Unlike mice, we are capable of turning inward and responding. Thus, whether we will end up like mice, or will build a better future for humankind is up to us. Let us make the choice to turn inward and respond. Let us learn to Dis-Solve Conflict from Within at its very source, instead of dealing with the myriad of escalating effects. Let us not focus on the rotting fruit, or even on the root. Let us start with the seed. The time is Now.

2

IT ALL STARTED
WITH A MOTORCYCLE

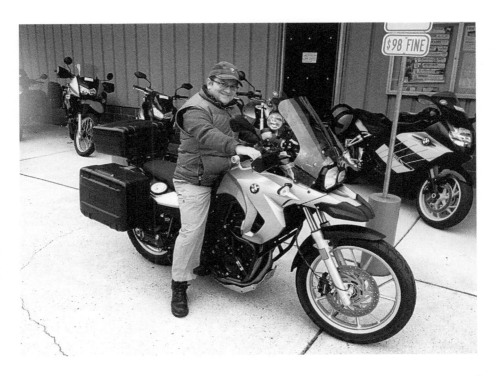

My own inner journey, which ultimately led to the creation of Dis-Solving Conflict from Within, began with a motorcycle. Motorcycles entered my life when I was a 32-year-old lawyer, working for a law firm in Philadelphia, specializing in personal injury and civil rights litigation.

Being a lawyer was an important, if not critical, facet of my identity. It satisfied my deep desire for connecting with people while serving them. It did not hurt that a career in law offered attention, power, prestige, and economic stability, all of which had eluded my immigrant family. I came to the United States in 1994 at the age of 14 along with my parents as a refugee from Ukraine. We came from Kiev, a large, relatively-cosmopolitan city, where my parents, an engineer and a nurse, enjoyed a mostly comfortable though increasingly unstable life. In fact, it was instability in the years which followed the break-up of the former Soviet Union; incessant anti-Semitism; and the probability of me being conscripted into the military at the age of 18 which drove my parents' decision to immigrate.

We emigrated to Scranton, Pennsylvania—a mid-size city in a coal-rich region of Northeastern Pennsylvania. Once Scranton was a bustling city with high-end stores and restaurants and even a highly active cultural, music, and Vaudeville scene. However, by the mid-nineties when we came, Scranton was in decline, joining dozens of rust-belt American cities which were past their prime.

Scranton's residents were mainly descendants of Irish and Polish immigrants who once worked the coal mines. There were few people of color and even fewer first-generation immigrants. In this environment, my fifty-seven year-old father, a mechanical engineer by training with very limited English proficiency, had few employment opportunities, and until he could no longer physically work, worked a series of menial, low-paying jobs. My mother, at the time a forty-four year-old nurse anesthetist, worked her way from a hospital housekeeper and nanny to a phlebotomist for the American Red Cross. My parents' combined income in America never exceeded $40,000.

As a fourteen-year-old student at Scranton High School, I had a hard time fitting in. While I excelled academically due to the rigorous schooling in Ukraine, the combination of my heavy accent; the culture shock of being in an environment completely foreign to me; and an embarrassment about my family's limited means translated into social awkwardness and very few meaningful connections. This changed, however, when I joined my high school's speech and debate team.

Over the years, in the quest for attention (and laughs), I often dramatized how I joined the speech and debate team. I frequently told a story of how I joined the speech and debate team by accident, after wanting to join the swim team and by being told that the swim team in English was called "speech and debate." While my English was hardly perfect at the time, I knew enough to know the difference between swimming and speaking. I joined the Speech and Debate team because Scranton's speech and debate program under the direction of Mrs. Eleanor Langnan had an almost cult-like status. Nearly every one of my teachers talked about the speech and debate program and many students in the Honors classes I took were part of it. So impactful and powerful was this program that my classmate and playwright, Stephen Karam, memorialized it in his award-winning, off-Broadway play called *Speech and Debate*.

Mrs. Elleanor Langnan, the head of the Scranton's Speech and Debate program, cut an imposing figure. In her sixties, with piercing gaze, intermittent Southern accent (she moved to Scranton from Tennessee), and the flamboyance of a former actress, Mrs. Langan single-handedly built Scranton's speech and debate program from scratch to one of the best such programs in the State and among the top in the nation. When Mrs. Langnan spoke, grown men trembled and teenagers did as they were told. There was no "else" with Mrs. Langnan.

Upon meeting me in all my 14 year-old, broken English glory, Mrs. Langnan ruled that I would be competing in Extemp. Extemp was shorthand for Extemporaneous Speaking—a speech and debate competitive category where one had to deliver a 5–7 minute speech on the topic related to current events after learning their topic exactly 30 minutes prior and thus having exactly 30 minutes to prepare. This was an odd category for someone just learning to speak English. It was also a stroke of genius. Mrs. Langnan made no mistakes.

I ended up loving public speaking! The thrill and pressure of thinking on my feet; speaking about topics that even grownups did not fully understand; opportunities to travel to speech competitions around the region, and later around the country; connections I made with other misfits, who spent their weekends at speech competitions; and the language proficiency and confidence I gained were all invaluable. It turned out I was good at extemporaneous speaking and since public perception of lawyering is so intricately connected with oral advocacy, I and those around me began to believe that I would be good as a lawyer.

Another important influence in my decision to become a lawyer was a realization of how powerless my parents were in the face of blatant bias against them. One incident stands out even after living in America for more than twenty-five years. About two years into our life in America my mom was fired from her job as a nurse's aide at a nursing home. She was accused of abusing a patient. This accusation came from another nurse's aide, a younger woman who has repeatedly mocked my mom's heavy accent and told my mom she was taking a job away from a qualified American. This woman and my mom were work partners and they were supposed to work together to take care of patients. Instead, the woman left my mom alone with a combative patient with late-stage Alzheimer's. The patient spat on my mom as she was trying to feed her. My mom, an experienced nurse, tried to pet the patient's cheek to calm her. The patient pulled my mom's hand away and scratched herself. My mom was alone with this patient at the time. Her work partner who was supposed to assist my mom was nowhere to be found. My mom was fired based on the word of her work partner. No one even bothered to ask my mom what happened. An immigrant woman was presumed to be at fault.

This incident really shocked our family. Not only was it financially devastating—at the time my mom was the sole breadwinner, but it was deeply painful for my mom who always prided herself in taking good care of others. Most importantly, however, it shook our until then unwavering faith in the inherent fairness and goodness of America. After this incident we became very cognizant of the plight of other immigrants and of Black and Brown people in this country, who faced systemic racism and discrimination in nearly every aspect of their lives.

By the time I entered college at the University of Scranton, I was set on becoming a lawyer and was doing all I could to prepare myself, including working as a paralegal for a small civil rights law firm and interning with the chambers of a local judge. Yet nothing prepared me for what I encountered when I actually became a lawyer.

My very naïve hope and idea was that as a lawyer I could empower, humanize, and protect people like my parents—poor, underserved, and often unnoticed. Indeed, these are the very types of people whom I represented as a civil rights, employment, and personal injury lawyer during much of my legal career. My clients' resilience in the face of most extraordinary challenges; their pain; their humanity and humility; their ingenuity; and their wisdom moved me deeply and were constant sources of inspiration and even awe for me. However, I was much less enamored with the legal process with which I was engaged daily and the impact it was having on myself and my clients.

The deeply ingrained pillar of the American system of justice is the adversarial process which culminates in the trial by jury. With some procedural differences, the adversarial process applies to both civil and criminal cases. At the core of the adversarial process is the idea that the best way to get to the truth and some semblance of justice is for each party to develop their case and then to present the case they developed to impartial fact-finders, namely the jury. The judge then acts as both the case manager and gate keeper. As case manager, the judge is responsible for shepherding cases through various stages of litigation. As gatekeeper, the judge decides what pieces of information actually constitute evidence. Evidence is what the fact-finder, the jury, actually gets to hear.

In reality, jury trials were too unpredictable, disruptive, and expensive and thus were extremely rare in civil litigation. Yet, lawyers like me spent most of their time preparing cases for trials. In this process, governed by complex, highly technical, and often arcane rules and traditions, lawyers and judges had extraordinary powers. Most cases were won and lost not in passionate arguments to jurors, but in voluminous legal briefs on often obscure and opaque legal technicalities. Another important aspect of litigation was discovery. Discovery is a process of obtaining and uncovering information that may be relevant to a lawsuit. It involves exchanging a series of written questions, production of documents and taking of depositions, the sworn testimony of witnesses. It was in discovery where I often saw the worst in lawyering—pettiness, obfuscation, grand-standing, intimidation, and downright bullying—all were very common tools. Also, the preparation of cases for trials involved reliance on a cottage industry of experts, investigators, and consultants, whose often highly inflated fees added thousands of dollars of costs to already very expensive cases. In rare cases which went to trial, many lawyers followed the advice of expert plaintiff's lawyer, Don C. Keenan and jury consultant, David Ball who in their book, *Reptile: The 2009 Manual of the Plaintiff's Revolution*, advocated appealing to the reptilian, most-primitive part of the juror's brain as a way to obtain large jury verdicts.[26] Translation—Keenan and Ball advocated scaring the jurors to death to maximize lawsuit recoveries. Still, most cases did not conclude in jury trials in ornate and dignified courtrooms with decisive and clear verdicts. Instead, they ended in drab conference rooms where lawyers, often without their clients and facing pressure and downright intimidation by judges, agreed to settle the cases. A good settlement, as one judge described, was a result where everyone was equally unsatisfied.

I found the whole thing fear-based, laborious, inefficient, ego-driven, and disempowering, especially to the poor and working-class litigants I mainly worked for. I became profoundly aware how acrimony inherent in litigation was destructive to relationships and basic human connections.

Binary, "us" vs. "them" thinking, inherent in an adversarial legal system, was bringing out the worst in me and in the attorneys and litigants I encountered. Positional arguments prevalent in an adversarial legal system did little to advance actual understanding between people. The parties, especially those of limited means, were swallowed by the system, which they did not understand, and which rarely gave them a voice or even cared about what was truly important to them. Courts serve an important function in our society and are necessary in many situations. Yet, it seemed like there had to be another less destructive and more wholesome way to deal with conflict. Soon, I would discover one.

Seven years into my legal career I felt bored, heavy, and unfocused. My grand visions of making Clarence Darrow-like closing arguments and empowering underprivileged clients collided with the reality of drafting motions in tedious discovery disputes and explaining to my clients why certain judges did not even bother making eye contact with them as they were pressuring me and them to settle their case. Like many of my colleagues I was perpetually frustrated, anxious, and drained by the practice of law. And I was desperate for a change.

It was then that motorcycles entered my life. Riding represented the passion, exhilaration, and freedom I craved. My newly found interest arose seemingly out of the blue, following a conversation with a rider friend. It was a surprise to everyone, including me. This newfound passion felt more like an obsession. To the great dismay and frustration of my loved ones, especially wife Juliya, I spent nearly every waking moment reading about motorcycles; looking at available ones on eBay; and taking steps towards learning to ride one.

Motorcycles became my vehicle for shifting my focus from outside of myself to within.

A few years before I began riding motorcycles, I learned Transcendental Meditation. My daily meditation practice was a source of solace which kept me centered in my hectic and increasingly frustrating life. Yet, it was riding motorcycles that took my mindfulness practice to a whole new level. Whether because of the inherent danger of riding; the skill and concentration it demanded; or the multitude of sensations that it brought; or perhaps because it was a radical thing for me, a short, stocky, bookish, conformist lawyer to do .When riding motorcycles, for the first time I experienced space between all the complex stories that were running through my mind and *me*. Even my identity as a lawyer, which was so central to how I saw myself, seemed to recede into the background. As a result, I felt more relaxed, focused, and at ease.

Motorcycles were also responsible for a critical meeting which quite literally put me on a different path in life. It was a beautiful spring day in Philadelphia, one of those days when the sun is shining but not burning, there is nary a cloud in the sky, and a light spring breeze lightly kisses the face. It was a perfect day for a motorcycle ride and I had every intention of enjoying this day on two wheels. Except that I woke up with strange pain in my lower back. Assuming it to be a pulled muscle, I hoped to walk it off. Yet the pain increased, soon becoming almost unbearable. A trip to the ER confirmed that I had a kidney stone. There was nothing to do except to wait to let the stone pass. Stuck at home, I was playing on Amazon, trying to find something to divert my attention away from the pain.

The movie I came across was called *The Highest Pass*. Produced by visionary director Adam Schomer, it tells a story of a young, Indian mystic and a Yogi, Anand Mehrotra, who took a group of Westerners on a harrowing motorcycle journey across the Himalayas. Riders, many of whom had limited experience riding motorcycles before the journey, confront manic Indian roads; deal with altitude sickness; and face their worst fears, all while being pushed to their limits and beyond by Anand. The point of the film is that the highest pass all riders have to climb is not in the snow covered, remote area of Northern India, but within them.

I felt deeply moved by this film and was fascinated by Anand. Just a few months later Juliya and I ended up meeting him at the Sattva Yoga retreat in Virginia. In person, Anand was just as irreverent and magnetic as he was in the film. His kind and penetrating eyes, with an ever-present twinkle, locked on mine as we came to greet him during the retreat. "You should come to India," he said, "and maybe you won't be so serious." He then burst into one of his frequent bouts of contagious laughter. That was the thing with Anand, with effortless ease he could switch from talking about the latest motorcycle model from BMW or Harley to explaining the nature of unconditional love, speaking with equal clarity, conviction, and captivation about both. One moment he was an innocent child, the next moment a sage. There was a dynamic stillness about him—bursting with energy, there was an undeniable fluidity and elegance about Anand apparent in his every action,from the way he walked and rode his motorcycle to the way he played harmonium while singing *kirtan*.

Not only were we fascinated with Anand, but the practice he taught, Sattva Yoga, which we were exposed to for the first time during the Virginia retreat, was also unlike any other yoga practice we had been exposed to before. Sattva, which translates from Sanskrit as 'whole,' combines elements of Kundalini, Kriya, Hatha, and Laya traditions of Yoga. We did not know any of this then. All we knew was that classes Anand taught combined meditation, breath, kriyas (yogic practices which combine breath with mantra and/or movement to move or awaken certain energies in the body), traditional yogic postures, and soft deliberate movement, similar to Tai Qi and Qi Gong. The effect on us was powerful. After the Virginia retreat, I felt clearer, more at ease, and more focused than I have ever felt in my life.

Because of the undeniable impact the retreat with Anand had on Juliya and I, we decided to accept Anand's invitation and travel to India. Since then, we have traveled to India thirteen times. In fact, in 2018, Anand and I, along with twenty motorcycle riders and twelve passengers, crossed the Himalayas together, retracing the original Highest Pass journey. Over the next eight years, Anand became my teacher and a very dear friend. Aside from my wife, Juliya, he has been the most influential person in my life.

I will not recount here many powerful and simply indescribable experiences I've had during my many visits to India. To unpack these experiences could take another separate book and then some. However, while in India I connected with the ancient Yogic teachings which are at the very core of this book. Fundamentally, while some spiritual traditions look up at the sky, or down at the earth, Yoga taught me to look within. An ongoing, life-long process of looking inward for answers has had the most profound impact on my life.

After my first month-long stay at the Sattva Yoga Center in the Indian holy city of Rishikesh, I came back to my law firm job in America feeling a bit discombobulated. My day-to-day work seemed so far removed from regimented, cloistered, and yet somehow inspiring and expansive life at a yogic ashram. Despite the powerful experiences I've had in India, I was not yet ready to give up the practice of law. However, I did feel inspired to explore different ways of being a lawyer. I also became much more cognizant of the mechanics of the day-to-day conflicts I was involved in. The possibilities of practicing law in a different way, as well as ideas of peacebuilding and conflict resolution, fascinated me and drew me in. My exploration exposed me to articles, books, and talks by lawyers Pauline Tesler, Stu Webb, Kenneth Cloke, Gary Friedman, Woody Mosten, J. Kim Wright, and David Hoffman which presented a tantalizing vision of lawyers as peacemakers. I felt especially inspired by "Collaborative Law," the law practice approach developed by Minnesota lawyer Stu Webb. Stu was a family lawyer in Minneapolis. Time after time he saw the unnecessary devastation the legal process brought to the families he was working with. Deeply influenced by the Eastern teachings on non-duality, Stu envisioned a different approach. After enlisting several like-minded colleagues, in 1998 he wrote a letter to the President Judge of the local family court. Stu's letter outlined an approach to family cases where lawyers at the outset of a case agreed not to proceed to court, instead focusing on working with each other and their clients to resolve the dispute. If the lawyers were unsuccessful, they would withdraw and pass the case to their litigating colleagues.

With the threat of going to court gone, parties and lawyers could share information and collaborate on working through whatever challenges the case presented. As there was no judge involved, lawyers could include the parties in meetings and schedule meetings at times actually convenient for families. Later on, Stu's model evolved to include at least one trained mental health professional to act as a neutral conflict coach for the lawyers and the parties. Starting with just a handful of lawyers in Minnesota, "Collaborative Law" became a worldwide movement, now with thousands of dedicated practitioners and many happy clients around the planet. "Collaborative Law" presented a possibility I could be passionate about!

On the way to becoming a collaborative lawyer, I had to become trained in mediation. That is how I ended up at the New York Peace Institute in the 40-hour mediation training, taught by Brad Heckman. Mediation felt like coming home for me as at the very core of the facilitative and trans-formative mediation models taught at the Institute was empowerment of the parties. In mediation, I found what I had been looking for for so long. I became committed to becoming the best mediator I could possibly be.

Becoming the best mediator I could possibly be meant that I had to dedicate my full-time efforts to learning this new discipline. With encour-agement from Anand, much self-reflection, and a heartfelt blessing from Juliya, I decided to quit my job at the Philadelphia law firm, where just a few months earlier I had been named a partner. Being a partner at a law firm, once a coveted dream, was no longer that important with my new inward focus. I decided to build a law practice fully dedicated to collab-orative law and mediation. Building such a practice meant that several times a week I commuted to New York from Philadelphia to volunteer as a mediator at the New York Peace Institute. I devoured every opportunity to practice my skills and took every training, including advanced mediation, group conflict dynamics, restorative justice, divorce mediation, youth-involved mediation, victim-offender conferencing, and conflict coaching that the New York Peace Institute offered. Eventually, I started working with some of the most difficult and intense conflicts and was invited to teach in the New York Peace Institute's prestigious apprenticeship program. This is how I discovered my love of connecting with people through teaching.

It turned out that a law practice focused on peacebuilding was a terrible business idea. People were so used to the image of lawyers as bulldogs! As a result, my law business tanked. However, I continued to hone my skills as a mediator, facilitator, and trainer. Organizations and individuals started retaining me more and more, not as a lawyer, but as a peacebuilder—a consultant who could help people deal with a range of complex conflicts in a more effective way. I found this work to be challenging, profoundly meaningful, and deeply rewarding. And, while I saw this work as consistent with the values and teachings of …, which were now so influential in my life, I was hoping to find a way to narrow the gap between the two even further. Life would show a way. Once again, motorcycles were involved.

As my personal mindfulness practice expanded significantly, riding was one way I could go even deeper within. And, yet again, motorcycles were responsible for another faithful meeting. At the invitation of my friend Bud Miller, a columnist for *Road Runner* motorcycle magazine, I started contributing to Bud's *Zen Motorcyclist* blog. One of my assignments for this blog was to interview Danish adventurer and author, Annette Birkmann. There were striking similarities between myself and Annette. Once, Annette was a successful lawyer in Copenhagen. Following a series of transformative events, which included a difficult divorce, Annette moved to Buenos Aires, Argentina. In Buenos Aires she became an assistant motorcycle mechanic at a busy motorcycle shop. Afterwards, Annette pursued her childhood dream and rode a motorcycle solo from Ushuaia, the Southernmost tip of Argentina, to New York. I loved Annette's book, *The Road to Getting Myself Out of the Way*, which was based on her journey, and I was excited to interview her. During the interview, I was struck by the clarity of Annette's insights, her humility, directness, and sharp wit. When we first spoke, I was still working at a law firm. Annette's audacity in quitting her job to pursue her dream was one of the inspirations for me to pursue mine. After the interview, it was apparent we had more to talk about. Over the next several months, we developed a very close friendship. It became very clear that something was emerging through us and that life was calling on us to work together. I invited Annette to become business partners with me and to work together on developing a mindfulness-based tool for dealing with conflict. To my amazement and delight, she agreed. It was through our collaboration that an early version of the Dis-Solving Conflict from Within process was born. Annette and I first shared this process with the public in Montreal, where at the time Annette was living with her partner. Sometime later, we taught together in Zurich. Both times we were astonished by the impact this process had on the people who participated in our workshops. It was clear that what emerged through us was much greater than us. Unfortunately, it also became clear that we had very different styles and priorities. While we valued and respected each other, we could not continue to work together. Annette left the company we had founded, The Living Peace Institute, and I stayed.

My work in conflict resolution continued to expand through The Living Peace Institute, which offered conflict resolution, organizational development, and executive coaching services around the world. I also felt extremely fortunate to continue to develop and share the Dis-Solving Conflict from Within process. Though, as I learned, running a business is not one of my strengths. When an opportunity came to join Virginia Tech's Office for Equity and Accessibility as the Assistant Director for Education, Outreach, and Conflict Resolution, I jumped at the chance. In this job, I get to do all the things I am deeply passionate about— teaching, coaching, mediation, and organizational development. It does not hurt that Blue Ridge mountains of Southern Virginia offer some of the best motorcycling roads in the world. I continue to be involved with The Living Peace Institute and India remains my second home.

While this book is about the Dis-Solving Conflict from Within process, it is also a culmination of all that I learned about conflict resolution from working with hundreds of complex conflicts in multiple settings around the world. This book is also a direct result of my own spiritual journey, though none of the materials in it require any particular set of beliefs. None of this would have happened, but for motorcycles.

3

THE ANATOMY OF CONFLICT

Conflict and Fire

I begin many of my workshops with a simple exercise. I divide the participants into three to five different teams, asking each team to come up with a name and a brief statement of what the team stands for. If there is time, I also invite each team to come up with a symbol which represents them. Once everyone comes back together, the spokesperson for each team shares their team's name, symbol, and values. Usually, the team names and symbols are clever and creative, and the values are both inclusive and aspirational. After all the teams finish, I pretend to fumble with my presentation. Then an ominous music begins to play. A lime green alien appears on the screen. "You measly earthlings!"—it says, voice full of contempt. "Enough of your nonsense! Your time has come!"—the creature continues. "We will destroy this planet unless you agree on one team which gets to survive. The choice is yours! The time is now!"—concludes the alien. Afterwards, trying my best to look frazzled, I inform the participants that our plans for the workshop have changed. I instruct them that teams now must negotiate with each other and present the participants with three Alien Rules of Negotiations: (1) No changing of team names; (2) No changing of team description; (3) If teams agree to merge, the merging team must give up its identity, assuming the identity of the surviving team. Grimly, I remind the workshop participants that the survival of the planet is in their hands, and as per the alien master's command the planet can survive *only* if the multiple teams merge into one, assuming the identity of that one team. I turn on the ticking clock, generally giving the teams fifteen to thirty minutes to negotiate with each other as I sit back and observe.

Almost inevitably the tension in the room rises as the teams frantically try to persuade each other to merge. Decisions often come down to the wire, with final mergers concluding as the buzzer rings. More than a few times I had to play a video of a mushroom cloud, symbolizing the failure of the teams to merge into one.

I learned this very powerful exercise from psychologist Dan Shapiro of the Harvard Negotiation Project who describes it in detail in his brilliant book, *Negotiating the Non-Negotiable*.[27] In fact, Dr. Shapiro conducted a much more elaborate version of this experiment at the World Economic Forum in Davos, Switzerland to a chilling result. With top world business and political leaders engaging in three rounds of intense negotiations, there was no agreement on the single surviving team. The world was destroyed!

This exercise/social experiment raises some very interesting questions. Considering that each team's values are generally aspirational and not mutually exclusive, why is it so difficult for the teams to merge? If the future of the planet was truly at issue, does it matter what the surviving team is actually called? Why is this tongue-in-cheek experiment, featuring a lime-green alien and ridiculous instructions, so triggering to the participants?

The answers to these questions offer profound insights into conflict. Before we consider the answers, let's start with some general observations regarding conflict. We treat conflict as the fire—this force outside of us we must avoid, escape, or control. The below drawing of a fire triangle reminds us of three elements of a fire—oxygen, fuel, and heat. I believe these three elements correspond with three critical components of conflict.

The oxygen in conflict is the story. In using the word "story," I mean the consistently persistent narrative we apply to life. Our story is a complex tapestry acquired and refined over generations. It consists of conditioning (the way we learned to react to particular stimuli; our cultural, religious, social, or professional background); our beliefs (thoughts we have carried with us for a long time, often through generations); our experiences (our interpretation of the events that took place in the past); and our projections and expectations (ideas and thoughts about other people and the future based on thoughts and ideas about the past). As we go through life, we continuously and often unconsciously build our story, as we pick things up through culture, books, television, and other sources of information we come in contact with. Our story is like the "software" which processes and gives meaning to the sensory and other inputs we receive.

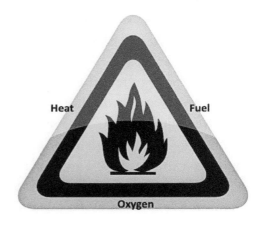

In the alien exercise, by coming up with the name, description, symbol, and values, each team has created a particular narrative. It was the second element of conflict which made this narrative so difficult to give up. Attachment is what turns our story from information, a collection of data, to *identity*, our perception that the story is *us*. In relation to our fire triangle, attachment is the fuel that makes the fire burn. Attachment to our story, or a sense of identity, is also what differentiates us from other people, giving us the sense of "us" and "them" as well as "*them*" vs. "*us*." Thus, our story and our attachment to our story are powerful forces in all conflicts because competing narratives, which challenge any aspect of our story, challenge something much more primal—our very idea of who we believe we are.

By the way, in referring to our identity as the story we are attached to, I don't want to diminish its importance in our lives. Stories are how we process life. Constructing a narrative is as ingrained in us as breathing. That is why stories are as natural, abundant, and essential as oxygen in our lives. Later on in this book we will talk about how just like we are not the oxygen that we breathe, we are not the stories running through us.

The greater the attachment to the story, the more rigid the identity, the more intense is the conflict which in any way challenges the story. After all, what would conflict between Israelis and Palestinians be if either side did not have a strong sense of attachment to their respective narratives? How would many divorce cases be different if one or both sides did not identify as victims, intent on avenging and punishing their partners? What would any of our conflicts, whether among co-workers or whole nations, look like without our narratives and our strong attachments to them? Also, once we are attached to a particular narrative, we enter a warp of sorts where our focus becomes very narrow, making us see life in diabolical, black and white, "us" vs. "them" terms. To illustrate this point, let's take a look at the below image. What do you see?

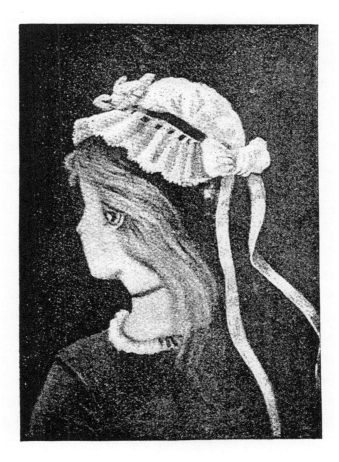

Do you see a young woman with her head turned away? How about a sad-looking old one? If this image was a conflict, wouldn't it be helpful for us to know if we are dealing with a young woman, a sad old woman, or both *before* we take action? Hence, this is why in our alien exercise the teams had trouble seeing that their respective values were not at all contradictory. And because of our ever-persistent narratives and our deep attachments to them, we never know the full story. In fact, most of the time we are looking at the world through a tiny keyhole of our own story, which of course includes our biases, conditioned beliefs, assumptions, judgments, and the like.

Coming back to our fire triangle analogy, the element we have yet to talk about is heat. In relation to conflict, heat is the movement of energy (e-motion) we experience when someone or something triggers us. This movement of energy, which some people actually experience as heat (hence the phrase "heat of the moment") are the experiences we label as anxiety, anger, frustration, and fear. In the West, and especially in the practices of psychology, psycho-analysis, and therapy we tend to focus on labeling and categorizing various emotions, forgetting that ultimately e-motion is both a visceral and multi-dimensional experience which alerts us to and reflects our inner state. In terms of the fire or conflict triangle, the movement of energy in the body alerts us to and reflects our triggered state. While ordinarily we have relatively little awareness of the story and the attachment to it (both oxygen and fuel are ever-present in nature to such an extent that we are not even aware of their existence), it is the e-motion or heat that serves as the most direct evidence of a fire letting us know that we are indeed in conflict.

As we look at these elements of conflict: story, attachment, and e-motion, an interesting question arises—where are all of these components residing? Aren't they all within us? Of course, there are people and circumstances which trigger us. They are like lit matches that light up the blaze. Yet, a match can land in gasoline or in water. The difference between the two, is the difference between *reaction* and *response*, which we will explore next. However, since all the elements of the fire we talked about are within us, what if conflict was actually not the fire we must avoid, escape or control, but a fire alarm, alerting us to what is happening within us.

Reaction and Response

By viewing conflict as the fire alarm, rather than the fire, by turning inward, we can learn to *respond* to it with strength, clarity, and ease, instead of *reacting* to it with fear, avoidance, or aggression.

In North America we tend to be very casual with our language, using the words "reaction" and "response" interchangeably. I suggest that these words have profoundly different meanings. Realizing the difference between reaction and response is critical for understanding our actions in conflict.

To better understand the distinction between the two, we need to take a brief look at neuropsychology of conflict. Our body perceives every trigger as a threat and makes no distinction on whether the threat comes from an impending attack by a lion or an obnoxious post on Facebook. Upon being triggered, the body activates its emergency system. As part of this activation, the brain activity transfers from the prefrontal cortex to the brain stem. The prefrontal cortex is the largest part of our brain, responsible for complex thinking and what we refer to as emotional intelligence—our ability to identify and empathize with the complex emotions of others. In contrast, our brain stem, also known as the reptilian brain, is one of the smallest parts of our brain. The brain stem is only concerned with survival and thus is only capable of fight or flight. Once activated, the brain stem directs the release of cortisol, a powerful hormone designed to mobilize and optimize our bodies resources for a life and death struggle or an all-in escape. The release of cortisol initiates blood and oxygen flow away from the brain and major organs to our muscles and extremities. Consequently, when triggered we become incapable of rational action and resort to conditioned and compulsive ways of addressing threats.

These conditioned and compulsive ways of dealing with threats are our re-actions in conflict. In other words, re-action is our attempt to control or escape whoever or whatever is triggering us. Re-action is the program that activates each time we are triggered. And the same re-actions repeat themselves time after time. Whether our "go to" re-action in conflict is to avoid, appease, escape, compromise, or attack, the core experiences are stress, doubt, and fear. When we re-act, our focus is outside of us, on whoever (or whatever) is triggering us. Re-action (even one we are not conscious of) is the product of deeply ingrained conditioning, experiences, beliefs, projections, and expectations. In other words, it is an integral part of our story. Sikh teacher and mystic, Yogi Bhajan put it best when he said:

> If you are willing to look at another person's behavior toward you as a reflection of the state of their relationship with themselves rather than a statement about your value as a person, then you will, over a period of time, cease to react at all.

Whereas a re-action by its very nature arises from a triggered or disturbed state, a response then is an action which arises from an undisturbed state. What differentiates the two is *where* the action is coming from. Having an undisturbed state requires some space between our story and us. Renowned Sufi poet Rumi beautifully illustrated this point when he wrote in one of his most famous poems: "There is a space beyond right and wrong…I'll meet you there." The space Rumi was referring to is the space where we can detach, however slightly, from our story. In that space instead of suppressing or expressing what is arising through us, we can observe it. In that space we go beyond thoughts. Awareness, Zen, Shunya are the words from different traditions which are used to describe this space. My word is very simple—peace. Response then arises from peace, from that place within us where we can detach and observe. Connecting with this space is what the Dis-Solving Conflict from Within process is about.

As all of this can get quite abstract, let me illustrate. A good friend of mine, "Rachel"[28] complained about an ongoing conflict with her son, "Michael." At the time, Michael was twenty years old and living with Rachel and her husband. As I know both Rachel and Michael well, I have had many opportunities to observe them together. It took very little to trigger Rachel. Seemingly anything Michael said or did provoked a reaction from her. She often snapped at Michael in public, criticizing and correcting him.

"Fixing" Michael was Rachel's life-long mission. But, Michael had little interest in meeting Rachel's expectations. When Rachel criticized him, Michael either snapped back with snarky remarks (triggering Rachel even further) or withdrew altogether. Even though Rachel and Michael lived in the same home and clearly loved each other, they began avoiding being in each other's presence as they simply could not communicate without fighting.

Rachel grew up in a strict home where her parents demanded perfection from their daughter. She was conditioned to be tough on herself and tough on others. The idea that Rachel knew what was right for herself and her family was deeply ingrained in Rachel's identity. Thus, whenever Rachel felt triggered, without even realizing it, she went to her "go to" reaction: to "fix" and criticize. Michael's reaction, in turn, was to attack Rachel back or to escape.

Rachel was open to going within and with my guidance she developed a regular mindfulness practice. Through this practice Rachel began observing herself in her conflicts with Michael. She noticed how the same reactions repeated themselves in different conflicts she had with her son and how deeply ingrained these reactions were within her. By becoming aware of her own conditioning, Rachel became more and more capable of noticing what was triggering her and responding to Michael instead of reacting. While Rachel and Michael still have some ways to go, they are learning to communicate and engage with each other in ways they have not been able to before.

In distinguishing re-action and response we have to be careful not to focus too much on what the outward action looks like, but rather, as the following example illustrates, where it comes from.

Lauren was a coaching client of mine who was going through a divorce with her husband. One day Lauren called me to ask my advice on whether she should resolve her divorce through mediation. Considering that I am passionate about mediation, serve as a mediator and train mediators,

Lauren could not find a better person to validate her desire to conclude her divorce through this process.

However, as Lauren and I spoke, it became clear that she was eager to seek mediation to avoid a confrontation with her husband. Avoidance is how Lauren reacted to conflict since the time she was a little girl. As Lauren and I worked through the Dis-Solving Conflict from Within process—quieting her mind, turning inward, and unconditionally feeling what is, it became clear that the appropriate response for Lauren was not to be the quiet lamb she always was. Rather, it was to roar like a lion. In this instance, the appropriate response for Lauren was to fight for herself.

Lauren's example illustrates an important point—response is doing what is needed in a particular situation from an undisturbed state of mind. Just as in life, an appropriate response could take many different forms and mimic all the five elements present in life. Sometimes the appropriate response is fire—to act with fierceness and intensity; sometimes it is earth—to ground and nurture; sometimes it is water—letting something flow away; sometimes it is air—to speak our truth; and sometimes it is ether—or to rise above the situation.

The *Bhagavad Gita*, the ancient Yogic text, provides one of the best illustrations of the difference between reaction and response. The text describes a dialogue between Arjuna, a prince warrior about to lead an army into battle and Krishna, the Divine who manifests as Arjuna's charioteer. Arjuna does not want to fight the opposing army, which consists of his cousins and other people he likes. He seeks Krishna's guidance on what to do. Curiously, Krishna does not advise Arjuna to abandon the battlefield and to hug it out with his cousins. Instead, Krishna tells Arjuna to get into Yoga first and then act from there. As the word "Yoga" in Sanskrit means "unity," Krishna is advising Arjuna to get into the state of unity within himself first, and then let the action arise from that place. That is the best illustration of a response that I have come across.

Space

If we want to stop the fire, we need to create space between oxygen and fuel. Likewise, if we are interested in transforming conflict, there must be space between us and our story. The concept of space is much misunderstood in the West as we associate it with disengagement, non-involvement, emotional distance, or worse, with apathy. Nothing could be further from the truth. On the contrary, space is *full* engagement but without the entanglement. It is the ultimate act of humility, a deep realization of how limited and biased our knowledge is. It is an innate awareness that regardless how compelling or meaningful our stories might be, we are not them. Space is like being in the movie theater watching a movie, as opposed to being in the movie. When we are in the movie, we lack the awareness that we are in the movie. Our re-actions to various actions and characters take over us. On the other hand, when we are in the movie theater watching the movie, we can be fully engaged in the action; we could sympathize with various characters, while experiencing a range of emotions. Yet, there is innate awareness that we are not the action on the screen; that while we may have a preferred ending, we did not write the script and thus the ending is not up to us; that while watching a movie, we could have our popcorn, and at the end of the movie, get in our car and leave. Cultivating space in conflict between our stories and us means we draw clear distinction between what is *us* and what is *ours*. This distinction is critical for responding, as opposed to reacting, to conflict and something we will be working on throughout this book.

Feeling Better

One of the key motivators for our reactions in conflict is the quest to avoid pain. But what if feeling pain was ok? What if we weren't so afraid of it? Being open to pain fully and unconditionally can become the very source of our liberation. In fact, it is only by connecting fully with our pain, not escaping it, that we can truly transcend it. Addiction and recovery expert Tommy Rosen addressed this very point in his brilliant book, *Recovery 2.0.* Tommy wrote:

> We imagine that the most horrible things will happen if we dig into the original hurts, but ironically, it is only by looking directly at the pain that we can begin to understand it, process it and heal it.[29]

American author and activist James Baldwin wrote poignantly about pain and its power to connect us with others:

> You think your pain and your heartbreak are unprecedented in the history of the world, but then you read. It was books that taught me that the things that tormented me most were the very things that connected me with all the people who were alive, who had ever been alive.

Annette Birkmann, the co-creator of Dis-Solving Conflict from Within, experienced a deep sense of freedom when she embraced unpleasant e-motions, instead of escaping them. In her book *The Road to Getting Myself Out of the Way* she wrote:

> If freedom doesn't include the possibility of feeling sadness, anger or fear, is it real freedom? No. It's living in fear that "bad" stuff might happen to me. But if there's no escape from the "bad" stuff, if the "bad" stuff is allowed, what can then truly hurt me? Am I not free? Yes, indeed I am.

If we are to transform conflict and learn to respond to it, we have to become comfortable with the discomfort of pain. If even pain is ok, what could truly hurt us? In fact, here I'd like to distinguish between pain and suffering. Whereas pain is our visceral experience that is integral in being human, suffering is our story about the pain. Pain is inevitable, powerful, and transformative. Suffering is optional. Through the Dis-Solving Conflict from Within process we will be intimately connecting with our pain, while creating some space between us and our suffering. In this sense, the Dis-Solving Conflict from Within process is not a tool for feeling better. Rather, it is a way to get better at feeling, feeling *all* that is arising within us. Feeling *all* fully and unconditionally without suffering is key to *responding* to conflict and to dis-solving all conflicts from within.

Part Two

DIS-SOLVING
CONFLICT FROM WITHIN

4

THE TOOL

So, what is Dis-Solving Conflict from Within? At its essence, Dis-Solving Conflict from Within is a simple, four-step process for turning our attention inward in conflict. The purpose for turning our attention inward is not to fix, label, or analyze our inner experience. Rather, the point is to unconditionally be with whatever is arising. Having the capacity to unconditionally be with whatever is, is how we develop space between us and our stories. As we discussed, it is this space which allows us to *respond* to conflict, instead of *reacting* to it. Once we learn the tool, it will become clearer how to use it. In fact, I invite you to read this chapter at least once all the way through and then come back and practice the tool.

The tool itself consists of a simple but powerful breathing technique, which is used as an anchor during the four steps of the process. Each of the four steps contain simple questions or affirmations. The purpose of these questions is to bring our awareness to various aspects of our conflict experience. We will begin by learning the Connected Breathing technique. I learned this technique from Michael Brown and his book *The Presence Process*.

Connected Breathing Technique

Breath is the simplest, most direct, and ever-present way to shift our focus from outside of us, within. That is why this breathing technique is an integral part of the Dis-Solving Conflict from Within process. To practice this technique, sit up tall with your spine comfortably erect. It is best to have your feet firmly planted on the ground. Gently close your eyes and notice your breath. Notice the colder air entering the nostrils and the warmer air leaving. Consciously make the breath deeper, allowing it to travel to and through the chest, the stomach, and even to and through the pelvic floor. As you breathe deeply, but without straining, pause as little as possible between each inhale and exhale. It may be helpful to picture pouring olive oil from one container to another, allowing the breath to move as oil—in one continuous and smooth flow. Next, we will introduce a simple, four-word phrase to help us tune-in. The phrase is: "I am here now." It is helpful to coordinate this phrase with the breath: as you inhale, think of the word "I"; exhale—"am"; inhale—"here"; exhale—"now." The brief description of this technique is below:

Connected Breathing Technique:

- Gently close your eyes and focus on the breath

- Inhale deeply, while exhaling completely

- Be sure to breathe with diaphragm and the stomach

- Focus on the inhales, allowing the exhales to just happen naturally

- Pause as little as possible between the inhales and exhales

- Let the breath move in one smooth continuous motion

- Use mantra: "I am here now" with the breath

- Inhale "I", exhale "am", inhale "here", exhale "now."

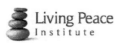
Living Peace
I n s t i t u t e

An MP3, guided version is available at: www.livingpeaceinstitute.com. Please, take a few moments to practice this technique right now and then reflect on your experience in the way that resonates best with you.

What did it feel like to practice Connected Breathing? It is not unusual for people who use this technique to report feeling calmer and a bit more spacious; it is also not unusual to experience physical or emotional discomfort, or even nothing at all. Whatever your experience, it was valid, complete, and just the way it needed to be.

There is an important reason why we utilize this technique. As we have discussed, our mind interprets conflict as a threat to us. Any perceived threat sends a signal to the reptilian brain, the smallest part of our brain located at the brain stem, to prepare for "fight or flight." "Fight or flight" is a primal human instinct, developed over thousands of years, to keep us safe. It involves the release of adrenaline and cortisol, the "fight or flight" hormones; sends blood and oxygen to our extremities and away from our brain; and makes our breathing very shallow. This primal instinct is incredibly useful for times when a wild animal is chasing us and our very survival depends on our ability to outrun it or overcome it in a physical fight. "Fight or flight" does not serve us so well in conflicts with loved ones, disagreements with bosses, and neighbor disputes. And it can have catastrophic consequences for groups of people and countries armed with sophisticated weaponry, including nuclear arms.

Connecting to our breath tells our body that an animal is not chasing us. Thus, instead of engaging the primitive brain stem, we activate the prefrontal cortex, the largest part of our brain. The prefrontal cortex is responsible for higher level thinking, such as analysis, planning, and relating to other people. Deep breathing also sends more oxygen to the brain, allowing our nervous system to relax. A relaxed, oxygenated nervous system translates into our ability to listen, empathize, and respond in conflict.

Breath is also what connects us with every living creature, including animals and plants, as what we inhale, they have exhaled and vice versa. Finally, breath is the link to the very intelligence of life—mechanically and chemically it is actually an incredibly complex process, a life-sustaining process, which life effortlessly takes care of for us. Wouldn't connection with this profound intelligence be helpful to us in navigating conflicts?

In fact, if you take nothing else away from this book, remember to breathe. In his book, *Stepping Into Freedom: Rules of Monastic Practice*, renowned teacher and Buddhist monk Thich Nhat Hahn said that: "Feelings come and go like clouds in a windy sky. Conscious breathing is my anchor." Consciously practicing Connected Breathing twice a day for just ten minutes could be absolutely life-changing. I invite you to give it a try! Connected Breathing as an integral and critical anchor of the Dis-Solving Conflict from Within process.

The Four Steps

The Dis-Solving Conflict from Within tool consists of four steps. The below diagram illustrates the four steps and their relationship with Connected Breathing:

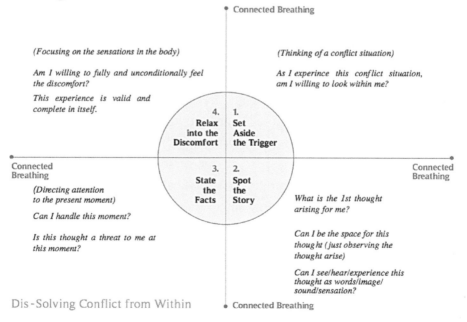

We will review both the rationale for and the mechanics of each of the steps of the tool.

Step 1—Set Aside the Trigger

The famous children's song and dance, Hokey Pokey begins with inviting the participants to "put their right leg in." The first step of the Dis-Solving Conflict from Within process is an invitation to look within. Practicing this step involves bringing the conflict situation into our awareness and asking—"With this situation arising, am I willing to look within me?" In posing this question, we are not suggesting that whoever or whatever has triggered us is not important. Rather, we acknowledge that we cannot control the outside factors, but can look within us to explore ways we could respond to the situation instead of reacting. It is important not to dwell on this question. As we pose it, the answer is the first thing that arises for us. If the answer is, "I am willing," we go on with the rest of the process, if it is "I am not," we stop after practicing a few rounds of the Connected Breathing technique.

Step 2—Spot the Story

The purpose of Step 2 is to spot the story that is arising for us in conflict and then to create some distance between us and the story. Spot means notice and observe. It does not mean analyze, change, or question. Step 2 of the process consists of two parts. In the first part we ask: "what is the first thought arising for me, as I experience this conflict situation?" Once we are able to spot the thought, we allow it to rise fully, without trying to analyze it or change it. The guiding question here is: "can I be the space for this thought?" In part 2 of step 2, we play a bit with the thought, to create some space away from it. We ask: "how is this thought arising?" If the thought appears as words, we spell the thought one letter at a time in front of us. If the thought arises as an image, we play with the image, making it larger or smaller. Finally, if the thought comes as sound, we manipulate the sound, making it quieter or louder. Sometimes, we cannot discern how the thought is arising. In that case, we could pick to play with the words, images, or sounds that are most closely associated with the thought. If there is a sensation associated with the thought, still work with words, images, or sounds. We will work with sensation in step 4.

Step 3—State the Facts

Step 3 of the process is about connecting with the present moment. The present moment is the only thing that we truly know as fact. Everything else, be it past or future, is just a story, which in fact does not exist anywhere outside of our head. Because much of our conflict experience is focused on past grievances or future anxiety, it is critical to come to the present moment and assess whether a conflict situation we are dealing with is truly a threat to us in this moment right here and right now. Another purpose of Step 3 is to empower us to handle this moment, regardless of what we may feel or what might be arising for us.

In practicing this step we bring our awareness to this moment, right here and right now. We then pose this step's two guiding questions: (1) "With this thought (the thought that we spotted in Step 2) arising, could I handle this moment, right here and right now? (2) Is this thought a threat to me at this moment?" In some ways, both of these questions are trick questions—the moment we asked if we could handle this moment, we already had. Thus, perhaps we could handle the next one as well. Likewise, very rarely (unless someone is suffering from PTSD) would a thought present an immediate threat to us.

This step really came alive for me following a motorcycle accident I had. One moment I was making a U-turn on a quiet, two-lane road in

Central New Jersey. In a split second, I was off my bike in a ditch, trying to comprehend what had happened. Only later I learned that I collided with another motorcycle, whom I did not see as I made my turn. As the initial shock of the impact wore off, a million thoughts started racing through my mind: "am I ok? What am I going to do? Did I break anything? How is the other guy and his passenger? Juliya will be terrified! How and why did I cause this accident? Will I ever ride again? Should I? What is life trying to tell me?" I focused on my breath and asked myself: "with all of these thoughts arising, could I handle this moment, right here and right now?" The answer was: "yes!" As I posed this question, I noticed my breath slow and my adrenaline-pumped body relax. I could move my arms and my legs. I then asked: "Are these thoughts a threat to me at this moment?" The answer was: "no." I relaxed even further and was able to pull myself up. The other rider and his passenger both came off their Harley, but were mostly okay. I could walk and was able to deal with the aftermath of the accident one breath at a time.

Step 4—Relax into the Discomfort

Step 4 of the process is the most important as in this step we connect with our e-motions. In connecting with our e-motions we first must ask the question: what is an e-motion? There is actually no agreement among scientists on what an e-motion is or how it arises.[30] Despite this, the definition that has emerged over the years is that e-motion is "a complex state of feeling that results in physical and psychological changes that influence thought and behavior."[31] As this definition suggests, e-motion is first and foremost a particular and very visceral experience. That is why I hyphenate the word e-motion to emphasize the experiential nature of it. E-motion is a movement of energy within us.

In the modern practice of therapy and psychoanalysis there is a significant emphasis on naming our e-motions. I don't find this practice to be particularly helpful, as it tends to reduce complex, multi-dimensional human experiences into words. These words often fail to capture the full depth and breadth of the experience they are supposed to describe. Sadness, anger, fear, and anxiety are all multi-dimensional experiences that include a multitude of sensations and experiences. Why reduce these powerful human experiences into words? Also, these words have a multitude of stories attached to them. Finally, through intellectualization and analysis, these words provide means to escape our e-motions, instead of actually *feeling* them. Thus, folks spend years in therapy analyzing and intellectualizing their e-motions, while actually just spinning their wheels.

I suggest that if emotions are an experience, what we call them does not really matter. It's like being in the rain. Whether we call rain *rain*, or *apples*, or something entirely different, there is an experience of rain that occurs. This experience includes the sensation of dampness in the air, the sound of rain droplets, the sensation of rain droplets hitting our skin, etc. Actually, by calling it rain we are reducing a multi-dimensional experience to something singular.

This is why step four is inviting us to connect with our actual experience, instead of our idea of that experience or our intellectual analysis of what that experience should or should not be. Thus, in this step we bring our attention to our body and focus on whatever we are experiencing as the thought (the story) about the conflict experience is arising within us. It is very important here to focus on the physical sensations regardless of how intense they might be (or even if they are barely discernible or not discernable at all). The guiding question in step 4 is very powerful: "Can I fully and unconditionally feel the sensation while knowing that this experience I'm having is valid and complete in itself?" The words "fully" and "unconditionally" mean that we are not trying to escape the pain or discomfort, but on the contrary are willing to embrace it fully. Yet we are also not allowing ourselves to go into a story about our experience. If we could unconditionally be with what really scares us or with whatever is arising for us in the most difficult conflict situations, aren't we taking back the remote from the individuals and circumstances which controlled us? If we could unconditionally experience anything (good or bad), isn't that a key to true personal freedom?

5

USING THE TOOL

Practice

Having talked about the elements of the process, we are now ready to put everything together into a cohesive practice. As you learn to use the Dis-Solving Conflict from Within process, it would be useful if you could find a space that is comfortable and quiet, limiting interruptions to a minimum. It would also be helpful if you could sit upright in a chair with some space between the back of the chair and your spine with your feet firmly planted on the ground. I recommend that you read the preceding chapter and the below instructions several times before practicing. You can also use a companion MP3 recording, which offers a guided version of the Dis-Solving Conflict from Within process. It is available at: www. livingpeaceinstitute.com.

A word of caution to those suffering from acute Post-Traumatic Stress Disorder, Clinical Depression, Multiple Personality Disorder, Schizophrenia or other mental health conditions: please consult with your mental health and/or health provider before practicing this process.

Begin the practice by bringing into your awareness (i.e. thinking about) the conflict situation you would like to work with. Don't try to analyze the situation, just bring it into your awareness as if watching a movie. It may be helpful to keep a notepad close by and to jot your situation down on it. Once the situation is firmly in your awareness, gently close your eyes and focus on your breath. Notice the cold air entering the nostrils and the warm air leaving. Consciously make the breath deeper, ensuring that it reaches the chest, the stomach, and even the pelvic floor. Consciously pause as little as possible between the inhales and the exhales, allowing the breath to move in one smooth, continuous wave. Gently introduce the focus phrase: "I am here now," remembering to coordinate it with the breath—as you inhale, think of the word "I", as you exhale, think of the word "am", as you inhale, think of the word "here", and as you exhale, think of the word, "now." Take a minute or two of just being with the connected breath and the "I am here now" phrase.

With your conflict situation in your awareness pose the first question: "With this situation arising, am I willing to look within me?" Just notice what answer is arising for you. Don't try to force a particular answer and don't think too much about it. Whether the answer is "yes" or "no," (i.e. "I am willing to look within me" or "I am not willing to look within me"), once again focus on the breath and practice a few rounds of the Connected Breathing technique. Only if you experience willingness to look within you continue on to Step 2. Otherwise, sit for as long as possible with your breath and then stop.

If you are willing to look within yourself, after practicing a few rounds of Connected Breathing pose the first question in Step 2—"As I experience this conflict situation, what is the first thought arising for me?" Notice whatever is arising in your awareness. It does not have to be particularly strong or coherent. Don't try to analyze the thought or argue with it. The key is just to notice what is arising for you. Once you've noticed the thought, pose the next question—"can I be the space for this thought?" Being the space for the thought means you are just observing it, as though watching a movie. Don't be afraid of the thought. It is just that, a thought. Let it rise fully!

After spending a few moments with the rising thought, notice how the thought is arising (i.e. is the thought arising as words, image, sound, or sensation). If the thought arises as words, spell the words one letter at a time in front of you; if it is an image you are seeing, play with the image making it bigger or smaller; likewise, with the sound, make it louder or quieter, perhaps picturing a little volume knob you are holding. If you notice the thought as a sensation, notice the sensation, but don't try to do anything with it. As we will be working with sensations in Step 4, use words, image or sound to express the thought. Pose the final question of Step 2—"Can I see/experience this thought as words/image/sound?" After noticing the answer to this question (whatever the answer might be), practice 3–7 rounds of the Connected Breathing technique.

Prior to starting Step 3, bring your awareness to the present moment. With your eyes closed, notice where you are sitting, your breath, and any other sensations happening in your body. Then pose the first question in Step 3—"With this conflict situation/thought arising for me, can I handle this moment?" Follow with the second question in Step 3—"Is this thought/situation a threat to me at this moment?" Continue with the process only if the answers to the above questions are respectively: "yes" and "no." If you do feel threatened by the thought and/or the situation at this moment, sit quietly, while practicing the Connected Breathing technique until the stress of the situation subsides. After completing the Step 3 questions, once again practice 3–7 rounds of the Connected Breathing technique before proceeding to Step 4.

As you proceed to Step 4, bring awareness to your body and focus on physical sensations that might be arising. Note, the body sensations may be very strong, barely perceptible, or there may be no discernable sensation at all. Regardless, focus on what is happening in the body as you pose the guiding question of Step 4—"Am I willing to fully and unconditionally experience the physical sensation/discomfort, while knowing that this experience I am having is valid, and complete in itself?" Continue to practice the Connected Breathing technique while staying with the sensation.

Don't try to fix it, analyze it, or make it go away. It is not unusual for the sensation to shift or change in some ways (i.e. become stronger or weaker). If the sensation shifts or changes, stay with the new sensation, while affirming—"This experience is valid and complete in itself." If you experience a new thought or the original conflict situation somehow evolves in your awareness, repeat the process. When repeating the process, skip Step 1 and start with Step 2 (i.e. "What is the first thought arising for me?"). Feel free to go through the process 3–7 times at one sitting.

While even one-time use of the tool could bring certain clarity to a conflict situation, regular use over time is what can unleash the real power of the tool, aiding the paradigm shift from focusing outside of us to turning within. Besides, sporadic use of the tool would make it very unlikely that it will be available in the moment during a truly stressful situation. Thus, my invitation is to use this tool every day for five to ten minutes, preferably in the morning for a period of forty days. You don't have to have an acute conflict situation to use the tool, it can be used with anything: persistent thoughts, daily annoyances, or just as a practice for observing anything that might be arising within us. Forty days is known as a mandala in the Yoga tradition. It is what it takes to establish and root a new habit. In fact, think of the Dis-Solving Conflict from Within process as the seed you are planting. That seed must take root, so that later on it can bear sweet fruit—the ability to respond to conflict with strength, confidence, clarity, and ease.

The Four Invitations

As you embark on the practice of the process, I would like to extend the following four invitations: (1) tune inward; (2) observe without evaluating; (3) expand; and (4) explore. As we will see later on, these four invitations have a much deeper dimension and play a critical role in conflict transformation. For now, we can think of these invitations as answers to questions why and how to practice the process.

The most important reason for practicing the process is to shift our focus from people and circumstances outside of us (most of whom/which we cannot control), to our inner experience. We spoke about tuning inward before; it is implicit in the name of the tool; and it is worth repeating again. Because tuning inward is a radical departure from how we usually deal with conflict.

My teacher, Anand Mehrotra, often says that "wherever we place our attention, that will grow." By placing our attention outside of us, we increase the relative importance of people and circumstances who trigger us. In essence we are giving them the remote control to our feelings and re-actions, allowing them to manipulate us as they see fit.

I was struck by the power we give away to the outside forces in one of the mediations I've handled. This case involved two senior business executives, a woman and a man, at a technology firm. While they had to work together, their relationship was quite toxic. The woman felt mistreated, disrespected, and side-lined by her male colleague. The man believed his colleague misunderstood her role within the company hierarchy and was not supportive of him. Over the course of three mediation sessions we were making slow but steady progress in charting the future course for these two individuals. That is, until the man used the analogy of the circus to describe their company. He said: "some people are ringmasters, they get to dance with the elephants. Others are there to pick up the poop." The implication of this phrase was clear: the man considered himself the ringmaster. The woman was deeply offended by this analogy and our mediation stalled.

Months later, the woman contacted me for conflict coaching. I learned that the man lost his job shortly after our mediation over his treatment of the woman, which she reported to the company's HR department. While the woman clearly won, she appeared sad and distraught when she came to my office for coaching. The misogynist male executive was gone, yet his offensive language continued to haunt the woman. She had trouble sleeping, had gained weight, and had difficulty focusing on her work. She reported that the analogy the man used, his taunting voice, and the smirk on his face as he used the metaphor was with her nearly every hour of the day. Even though he was no longer with the company, the man continued to exercise control over the woman.

Of course, the man's words and actions in the above example were disrespectful, deeply offensive, and inexcusable. However, by focusing on him, the woman gave away her power to him.

By tuning inward, using the techniques in this book, we grow our capacity for seeing the bigger picture and not letting other people's ignorance be as bothersome to us. It does not hurt also that through the Connected Breathing technique we send more oxygen to our brain, physiologically making it more inclined to reason, connect, and empathize.

As we start the process of tuning inward, the next invitation is to learn to observe without evaluating what is happening within us. This seemingly simple invitation can present an immense challenge in the world where judgments, evaluations, labels, and conclusions are the norm. Yet, learning to observe what is arising within us—seeing the symptoms, without the need to put a diagnosis or a label on our experience—is critical for creating space between our story and us, and thus for shifting from reacting to responding.

Expansion is the ultimate purpose and goal of the Dis-Solving Conflict from Within process. Thus, if we walk away after doing the process knowing something about ourselves and/or the conflict situation we didn't before, the process was a resounding success. Expansion also means that we realize how little we actually know. Our knowledge, regardless of how extensive, is always going to be limited. Our ignorance, on the other hand, is boundless. By working on creating space between us and our story, we are also quite literally working on expanding our awareness connecting with the transformative discomfort of not knowing, rather than the false and arrogant idea of knowing. Expansion also means letting go of attachment to any particular outcome. This is quite challenging, as letting go of the outcome requires us to accept the possibility that we do not know the full picture. It requires us to let go of the illusion of control. Yet this is also quite transformative, as it opens us up to the possibility of exploring solutions and outcomes we could not foresee.

Exploration is both a way to approach the Dis-Solving Conflict from Within process and the goal of using the tool. It is an invitation to have the courage to be curious. Whereas fear closes us, curiosity creates an opening. To paraphrase Walt Disney, curiosity keeps us moving forward, exploring, experimenting, and opening new doors. I believe the attitude of curiosity is essential to true conflict resolution. It is also key to Dis-Solving Conflict from Within.

As we begin exploring the tool, let us adopt the attitude of a baby learning to walk. When the baby takes her first steps, walking feels unnatural and awkward. She has to try things out and learn what it takes to keep her balance. There is a natural curiosity that drives babies to continue trying to take steps, even after a few possible hard landings on the butt. Babies have not yet learned about our ideas of perfection expressed through the harmful phrases like: "anything worth doing is worth doing well." If babies had that attitude, they would never learn to walk and would give up after the first try, announcing to the world that they are not good at this walking thing.

We need to adopt a different attitude—anything worth doing is worth doing *fully*, regardless of how many times our butt may hit the floor. Learning this process is not about becoming "good" at it (whatever that might mean), but rather engaging fully with each of the steps. As we practice Dis-Solving Conflict from Within, we may or may not see immediate results. If we can approach this tool with curiosity, while practicing tuning inward, observing without evaluating and focusing on expansion, while maintaining a playful and curious attitude of exploration, the results will come. We will be well on the way to Dis-Solving Conflict from Within.

Frequently Asked Questions

Question: So, what exactly are we trying to accomplish by using the tool?

Answer: First, we are creating some distance between our story in conflict and us. This distance is what allows one to be able to respond to conflict as opposed to reacting to it. Second, we are learning to connect with and experience our e-motions. As we will learn in later chapters, that is the key to learning how to communicate with others in a non-violent way. Third, we build resiliency, as now we know that we could face anything regardless of how difficult, challenging or unpleasant it might be. Fourth, we learn that we are not our stories or emotions. Thus, we realize that whatever we experience, does not have to define us. All of these open us up to be able to approach life's conflicts consciously and move through them with relative strength, clarity, and ease.

Question: Are we supposed to be using this tool before, during, or after a conflict situation?

Answer: Yes! The tool is useful in all stages of conflict. It is most important to form a habit of using the tool on a regular basis. This is why we recommend starting to use the tool for 10-15 minutes per day, daily for 40 days. There is no need to apply the tool to any particular conflict situation. Rather, it can just be used to engage with and process daily stressors of life. Forty-day daily use of the tool integrates the tool into our psyche and enables us to utilize the tool at times when we are particularly stressed or triggered.

Question: How do I know that I am practicing the tool right?

Answer: If you are going through the steps in the order in which they are written and are noticing different aspects of your experience, based on the prompts, you are doing it right. Please, be mindful of not getting lost in the head, trying to analyze your experience. Remember, this is a new paradigm, a new way to approach conflict. It will take some time to be able to integrate and use this new knowledge. Relax, take it easy, explore and expand.

Question: Am I supposed to feel something as I am using the tool?
Answer: Whatever is arising (or not) is absolutely OK. In fact, part of the invitation of the tool is to be OK with whatever *is*, whether the expression of *is* is subtle, dramatic, or even not there at all. Some people may have very vivid or even dramatic experiences, others may experience sensations that are very subtle, or even not feel much at all. All of these experiences are completely valid, complete, and appropriate in themselves.

Question: Is the tool appropriate for someone suffering from PTSD or another mental health condition, such as anxiety, bi-polar disorder or depression?
Answer: While the tool can be practiced by anyone, it is of critical importance that those suffering from any mental health condition practice the tool under strict supervision of their mental health and medical providers.

Question: What has been the experience of people who have been utilizing the tool?
Answer: Below is a sampling of reviews from people who have attended the Dis-Solving Conflict from Within seminars around the world:

Julie Carmalt, Ph.D. an academic at Cornell University wrote the following note to me after using the process:

I am writing to let you know of the marvelous shift that has occurred since participating in your workshop. I have had so many opportunities to practice dis-solving conflict and living with a peaceful and open heart. I have found my 'sacred pause' that seemed to have been missing. I feel a sense of space within from which I can pause, breath, reflect and let go. It is glorious and I'm so grateful.

Christine Kiesinger, Ph.D. an academic and communications and wellness expert wrote after participating in the Dis-Solving Conflict from Within seminar:

> It is my highest wish that everyone on the planet could take this training. I am convinced that when one understands that the first step in managing conflict is going 'within,' we could create world peace. Truly, this approach is innovative and turns current paradigms of conflict upside down. The content is invaluable in one's relationship to Self, significant other and work life. I look forward to honing my skills.

Another seminar participant and business owner, Kim Bucari observed:

> The Dis-Solving Conflict from Within seminar made me see myself and my role as a human being in a whole new light. As a participant in the universe, not just my finite little world. I gained invaluable knowledge on how to remove conflict as something personal and put it outside myself in order to deal with it in a positive manner.

Mental Health Counselor, facilitator and law student, Greg Gilston shared his experiences with the process, stating that:

> The Dis-Solving Conflict from Within process opened my eyes to a fascinating new method of feeling, experiencing, and being. This seminar was so intriguing, so valuable for anybody who wants to explore themselves from the outside looking in!

Corporate trainer and process user Jason Preat agreed:

> This process is a very powerful tool to dissolve internal conflict. It is elegant in its simplicity and can help you unearth deep feelings and release them.

Finally, Steven R. Covey endorsed author and internationally-renown conflict resolution expert, Stewart Levine described his experience with the tool as follows:

> The Dis-Solving Conflict from Within process gives you the tools to move through conflict on an energetic level. Subtle in its application but powerful in its impact the letting go generated has ripple effects that make a great contribution to resolution.

Part Three

TRANSFORMING CONFLICT

6

OURS AND US

Inspired by the film, *The Highest Pass*, and by the teachings of Anand Mehrotra, in the summer of 2018 I traveled to India to participate in a motorcycle journey to and through the highest motorable road in the world, the highest pass in the Himalayas. This motorcycle adventure retraced the journey depicted in the 2012 film, which had such a profound impact on my life. Anand's intention for our group of thirty-two was to experience the mystical aspects of existence and to go beyond the limitations of the body and the mind.

I am not sure what my personal intention for the journey was, other than to surrender fully to the experience and to survive. I also thought this journey would provide a diversion from what became my full-time work—peacebuilding and conflict resolution. Little did I know that this motorcycle adventure would offer powerful insights for my work.

In many ways, riding a motorcycle through the Himalayas was like being in an intense personal conflict. Narrow mountain roads without guardrails, maddening traffic, sixteen-hour days in the saddle, wild temperature variations, altitude sickness, mental and physical fatigue, as well as tensions among the colorful characters which comprised our group of thirty-two threatened and triggered me in the ways I've never been threatened or triggered before. In the below image my dear friend, Claire Zovko, captured the grit it took to traverse just one muddy mountain road on the way to a high-altitude city of Manali in the state of Himachal Pradesh (you can see me in my bright yellow helmet in Claire's rear view mirror).

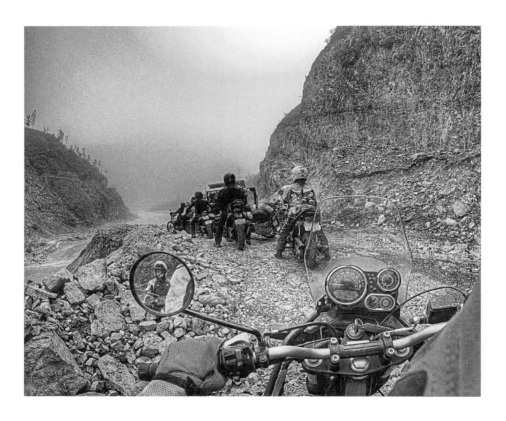

I *reacted* to being triggered by trying to escape, avoid, or control what I perceived to be my triggers. Briefly, I considered walking away from the journey and getting on the next plane to the U.S. But I had waited so long to do this journey, walking away would be a choice I would regret for the rest of my life. I decided early on that quitting was not an option, so I stuck with it. Sticking with it meant that I rode as slowly as possible, maintained a death-grip on the handlebars, and looked just in front of my front wheel. At the same time, my mind played an endless reel of *coulds* and *shoulds*. If you know anything about being on two wheels and especially when riding roads which would challenge even expert off-road riders, these are the worst possible things you could do. And, if you know anything about being human, the *coulds* and the *shoulds* could make us miserable even in paradise.

Yet, with every mile, every hairpin turn, every high altitude pass, every night spent under clear, mountain skies, something profound was changing within me: I was tuning more inward, becoming more aware of my experiences; I was evaluating less, and observing more; I was realizing how little I knew about anything, including even who or what I was; and I was becoming more and more curious about everything I was seeing in front of me. At the same time, my preferences, beliefs, thoughts, impressions, information, and even the needs of the body were becoming less and less important. The higher we climbed, the more at ease, focused, and present I felt.

The culmination of the journey for me was reaching the Khardung La Pass, which at 18,350 feet above sea level is as far and as high as you could travel on a motorcycle in the Himalayas. On so many levels, standing on top of the Khardung La Pass felt deeply profound.

First, I felt out of my mind. Past experiences, impressions, judgments, and memories, which make up what we call our mind, could not grasp or comprehend the sheer magnitude, raw beauty, and dynamic stillness of what I was seeing in front of me. So, at least for a bit, the mind went quiet—it did not have a label, judgement, evaluation, or a conclusion to put on the experience. Second, I was absolutely in the moment, observing and accepting it fully just the way it was. Finally, I felt really, really small. Standing at over 18,000 feet and realizing that Everest is another 10,000 feet up made me feel like I was the tiniest micro-speck of dust. My beliefs, preferences, roles, likes and dislikes, and personal story felt like distant stars in the mountain skies. With a quiet mind, being absolutely present, and distant from all the things that made up my identity, I felt more attuned and connected to everyone and everything around me in ways I have never felt before. Mine and my fellow travelers' eyes welled with tears. Small annoyances, minor squabbles, and even major differences that arose among us during this journey all dissolved into this moment. We didn't need words to feel so connected as not being able to tell where one person ended and the other one began.

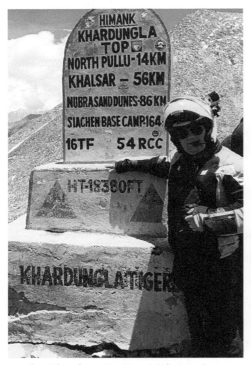
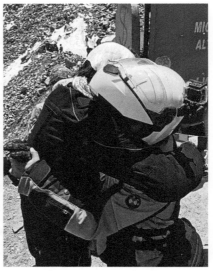

At the Khardung La Pass Mile Marker   *Embracing Anand at the Highest Pass*

The Khardung La Pass was not the end of our journey. However, the way that I rode and responded to challenges on the road changed. A life and death struggle became a dance. Clearly, I survived and my experience at the top of the Khardung La Pass fulfilled my teacher's intention for this journey. Experiencing this level of connection for me felt mystical and certainly took me beyond what I thought of as my body and my mind.

I realized that all the things I thought were *me* were accumulations: this body was an accumulation of food; this mind wasan accumulation of impressions, beliefs, judgments, prejudices, narratives, and information. So, what I thought was *me*, was actually *mine*. This realization, in turn, opened me to an insight about human connection. I discovered that these accumulations, regardless of how unique, similar, or interesting, are not how we truly connect with each other. I felt the most connected when all of these accumulations were the least relevant and the most distant. So, we connect with other people not through our identities but through something much greater and deeper.

In fact, I began to see our identities as boundaries. Like all boundaries, they work in some contexts, for a while, they can define and protect us, and create an illusion of separation, an idea that there is *you* and *me*, and *us* and *them*. Eventually, though, our identities, like all boundaries, enclose, limit, and confine us. Thus, the key to true connection and to transforming conflict is to go beyond these boundaries, or at least to make them a bit less rigid and defined. When we are able to do that, we discover space for connection that is truly profound, for connection which goes beyond beliefs, judgments, prejudices, similarities, likes and dislikes, and even beyond this physical form. It is this realization that has had a powerful impact on my work. Creating some space between *our* identities and *us* is how we transform our conflict interactions.

I suspect that this is a point in the book where some readers may get very angry with me. "How dare I—a white, cis-gender male, empowered by my privilege to do self-discovery adventures through the Himalayas, make broad pronouncements about identities like the one above???" "How are marginalized communities—people ostracized based on their race, color, national origin, disability, gender identity, gender expression, sexual orientation, or socio-economic status supposed to create space between *them* and their *identities*???" "Don't their identities not only define who they are, but also define their experiences and interactions with the society at large???"

I would still argue that identities are narratives we take ownership of, thus they are *ours*, but are not *us*. I am not suggesting here that someone's race, sexual orientation, or gender identity is a narrative. However, I am suggesting that the meaning we assign to these characteristics *is* a narrative which changes depending on the circumstances, our surroundings, and prevalent implicit and explicit narratives at the time. For instance, being Black in America and Black in Eritrea carry very different narratives. Likewise, identifying as a twenty-first century woman in Europe carries a different narrative than was being a woman in nineteenth century Russia. Even at different points in our lives some narratives are more prevalent than others. For instance, a young child may identify very strongly as a member of a particular family, while her narratives of race, gender, national origin, gender identity, and sexual orientation might not be as dominant. However, as the child grows into young adulthood and begins to be more impacted by societal narratives and discovers her role in the society at large, her race or sexual identities may become more important. As the young adult enters adulthood, role and career based narratives may prevail. Thus, this person may identify as a college professor, mother, and a partner more so than she identifies as bi-sexual, Latinx or by being originally from Chicago. As the same person progresses towards older age, prevalence of different narratives may again shift where narratives of familial roles, personal and professional accomplishments, and connection with a particular locale may dominate over other identities.

In Part II of this book, when discussing conflict in terms of a fire triangle, we talked about the role the story or narrative and our attachment to it plays in conflict. The biggest concern with the story is that our stories and thus our identities (stories we attach to) tend to be binary—victor/victim, good guys/bad guys, them/us. As the *New York Times* columnist, Ezra Klein noted in his book, *Why We Are Polarized*, sorting into rigid binary identities is at the very core of our current polarization as a nation. With binary identities conflict is inevitable.

It is actually incredible how quickly we form identities—get attached to a particular narrative and then start seeing the world in binary, *us* vs. *them* terms. Social Psychologist Henri Tajfel proved this very point in his famous Social Judgement Theory Experiment.[32] Tajfel and his colleagues showed twelve paintings—six by Paul Klee and six by Wassily Kandinsky to a group of forty-eight teenage boys, asking them to identify the paintings they preferred. Klee and Kandinsky were early twentieth century painters who produced very similar abstract paintings. The researchers did not tell the boys which one of the painters drew the particular painting, but divided them into groups, telling the teenagers that the group divisions were made based on their artistic preferences. In fact, the group assignments were random. Although the boys knew each other socially prior to the experiment and thus had multiple other social alliances among them; once allocated to one of two groups, they began seeing each other as either fans of Klee or Kandinsky. When researchers asked the boys to anonymously allocate rewards to other boys, despite the fact that actual group allocations were random and arbitrary, the boys showed clear favoritism towards "their" group and clear prejudice towards what they perceived as the "other" group. I've observed something quite similar when going through the Alien Exercise, described in Part II of this book. After creating a team description in the matter of ten to fifteen minutes, it was remarkable how much affinity people felt with their team and how difficult it was for them to give up their identity, even if giving up their identity meant saving the world.

Sport fandom provides another colorful illustration of the power our identities hold. Although affinities towards one sports team vs the other are often based on completely arbitrary factors, such as the team's affiliation with a particular geographic locale, many people see sports rivalry in life and death terms. Writer Will Blythe dedicated his book, *To Hate Like This Is to Be Happy Forever* to the meaning and intensity the rivalry between the University of North Carolina and Duke basketball teams brought to his life, tellingly writing: "[t]he living and dying through one's allegiance to either Duke or Carolina is no less real for being enacted through play and fandom."[33] As arbitrary and superficial our sports-related identities can be, for some they are matters of life and death.

Perhaps foreseeing the danger of rigid, binary identities, even America's founding fathers, George Washington, Thomas Jefferson and John Adams rallied against political parties. In his Farewell Address to the Nation, Washington said:

> [Political parties] serve to organize faction, to give it an artificial and extraordinary force; to put, in the place of the delegated will of the nation, the will of a party, often a small but artful and enterprising minority of the community; and, according to the alternate triumphs of different parties, to make the public administration the mirror of the ill-concerted and incongruous projects of faction, rather than the organ of consistent and wholesome plans digested by common counsels, and modified by mutual interests. [...] **Let me now [...] warn you in the most solemn manner against the baneful effects of the spirit of party.**[34]

In a letter to a friend, Francis Hopkinson, Jefferson wrote:

> I never submitted the whole system of my opinions to the creed of any party of men whatever in religion, in philosophy, in politics, or in anything else where I was capable of thinking for myself. Such an addiction is the last degradation of a free and moral agent. **If I could not go to heaven but with a political party, I would decline to go.**[35]

And, Adams noted in one of his letters:

> **There is nothing which I dread so much as a division of the republic into two great parties,** each arranged under its leader,

and concerting measures in opposition to each other. This, in my humble apprehension, is to be dreaded as the greatest political evil under our Constitution.[36]

My experience of riding a motorcycle through the Himalayas was so challenging on so many levels and so different from all the prior experiences that I've had, that it did not neatly fit into binary narratives I carried. Thus, my various identities were collapsing, or at a minimum, expanding. As my fellow travelers were going through a similar experience, our collapsing stories and identities created a powerful bridge for us to connect on. This is very common for people who go through powerful experiences together. For instance, many New-Yorkers, hardly a group of people known for being particularly warm and fuzzy towards each other, reported forming spontaneous and powerful connections in the immediate aftermath of 9/11. Likewise, when the Tsunami hit the South of India and thousands of people literally lost everything, people were able to simply serve their fellow humans. In all of these situations binary identities collapsed as they did not fit into the mind's typically binary paradigm.

Changing the binary paradigm means that even for a split second we must experience ours and other people's identities as fluid, flexible, nuanced, and expandable narratives rather than constant, rigid, and defined descriptors of who we are. In other words, we must expand our identity to include more than a very limited idea of *us*. Once we are able to do that, the idea of *us* and *them* will collapse. Once this idea collapses, conflict is transformed. In transformed conflict there may still be profound differences and disagreements. However, with the differences and disagreements there is room for immense growth, powerful connection, and meaningful dialogue.

In my work with many complex conflicts, I found four key principles to be at the core of conflict transformation. These principles and the practices associated with them move conflict from the one based in identity, domination, and rigid ideas of "right" and "wrong" to an exploration in shared humanity, expansion as well as complexity and nuance. These four principles are: tuning inward, observation without evaluation, expansion, and exploration. These principles are at the core of the Dis-Solving Conflict from Within process and are essential for living from within. It is these principles that have the power to transform most conflict interactions. Coming to think about it, what made my motorcycle journey across the Himalayas so transformative were these four principles which were ever present throughout my journey: tuning inward, observation without evaluation, expansion, and exploration. We will be exploring each of these principles and the practices which flow from them in detail in the following chapters. Then, in Part IV of the book, we will talk about three powerful conflict resolution methodologies: compassionate communications, restorative approach to conflict, and mediation. The four principles: tuning inward, observation without evaluation, expansion, and exploration are both at the core of these methodologies and are also their ultimate goals.

7

TUNING INWARD

The Purpose of Tuning Inward

In the Yoga tradition, the teaching of Ahimsa, or non-violence, is one of the most important. According to Patanjali, a prolific sage from 3rd Century BCE who authored one of the most important works on Yoga, *The Yoga Sutras* by Patanjali, Ahimsa is one of eight limbs of Yoga. Despite its relative importance, Ahimsa is easy to overlook as one can assume that they are living in a non-violent way by generally being kind to other people, caring about the environment, and supporting the right social causes. Another faulty assumption is to equate Ahimsa with pacifism. There is a lot more to Ahimsa than the perennial Golden Rule, a woke Instagram feed, or a dogmatic, and thus inherently violent, commitment to always turning the other cheek. At its core Ahimsa is about developing full awareness of our propensity for violence. As Anand Mehrotra often points out: there are only two types of violent people—those who have not been triggered enough to be violent and those who are aware of their violent nature and are doing something about it. In that sense, Ahimsa is not about what form an outward action takes, but rather is about what is behind the action.

Behind many of our actions is the very dangerous, violent, faulty, and ever-present idea of separation. Namely, that there is a separate and distinct "you" and a separate and distinct "me"; and that we are separate and distinct from nature and all that we interact with and all that surrounds us. This idea is at the core of the binary, rigid identities we tend to sort ourselves into and the binary "us" vs. "them" thinking we talked about earlier. So prevalent and persistent is this way of seeing life that it is a trap each and every one of is highly susceptible to falling into.

In her brilliant book, *High Conflict: Why We Get Trapped and How We Get Out*, Journalist Amanda Ripley illustrates how easily one of the world's most experienced peacebuilders fell into this trap. Ripley shares the story of Gary Friedman. Gary is one of the forefathers of the modern mediation movement. In his many workshops and writings he emphasizes the transformative nature of understanding in conflict. Gary has also traveled around the world teaching a form of active listening called looping. Finally, Gary is a practicing Buddhist and an experienced meditator. While I've not studied with Gary directly, his teachings have had an enormous influence on me and are an inspiration for my work. Yet, when Gary ran for a minor, volunteer political office in his small community in California, he quickly fell into the "us" vs. "them" trap. As Amanda Ripley describes, it took enormous effort, including a considerable amount of meditation for Gary to extricate himself from this trap. I did not lose any respect for Gary after reading about his experiences with high conflict. On the contrary, I respected Gary even more and I could totally relate to Gary's experiences. I do this work for a living and spend hours each day in my own practice, yet sometimes all it takes is a poorly timed social media post to trap me.

One of the key ways we express our violence and the idea of separation is through exclusion. Social Psychologist Kipling Williams has dedicated his life to studying the impact of exclusion and ostracization. In one of his most famous experiments, a person would be invited to play ball with two other people. At first all three people would toss the ball to each other. Then, two people (who actually were instructed by the researcher to start excluding the other) would start doing just that—tossing the ball to each other, but not to the invitee. When that happened, inevitably the excluded person experienced distress. This happened even when the excluded person was fully aware of the point of the experiment or even when the experiment ran virtually as a computer simulation. Despite the known negative effects of ostracization and exclusion, exclusion and ostracization are at the very core of many of our social, political, cultural, and educational structures.

Another way we express our violence is through contempt. Contempt is the ultimate act of violence as it creates a grotesque caricature out of a human being, denying that being's very humanity. Thus, contempt turns a being into a thing, unworthy of respect and deserving of cruelty and ridicule. So toxic is contempt that renowned relationship researchers John and Julie Gottman called it the "sulfuric acid" of a relationship. In their research the Gottmans studied thousands of couples and could predict with near mathematical certainty which couples would stay together and which would not by watching just a few seconds of the couple's interactions. Nearly always when the Gottmans detected the presence of contempt, the relationship was doomed to failure. American social scientist and *Washington Post* columnist Arthur C. Brooks sees contempt as one of the greatest threats to the American political discourse. In his book, *Love Your Enemies: How Decent People Could Save America From the Culture of Contempt*, Brooks wrote:

> We don't have an anger problem in American politics. We have a contempt problem. [...] If you listen to how people talk to each other in political life today, you notice it is with pure contempt. When somebody around you treats you with contempt, you never quite forget it. So if we want to solve the problem of polarization today, we have to solve the contempt problem.

In many of her books and talks, best-selling author, TED speaker and shame researcher Brené Brown talks about the dangers of scarcity thinking.

I believe scarcity thinking is one of the most destructive ways we express our violence. Scarcity thinking is a continuously perpetuating myth that we are not enough. Humanitarian and best-selling author Lynne Twist brilliantly captured the scarcity thinking phenomenon in her book, *The Soul of Money: Transforming Your Relationship with Money and Life*. She wrote:

> For me, and for many of us, our first waking thought of the day is 'I didn't get enough sleep.' The next one is 'I don't have enough time.' Whether true or not, that thought of not enough occurs to us automatically before we even think to question or examine it. We spend most of the hours and the days of our lives hearing, explaining, complaining, or worrying about what we don't have enough of. [...] We don't have enough exercise. We don't have enough work. We don't have enough profits. We don't have enough power. We don't have enough wilderness. Of course, we don't have enough money ever.
>
> We're not thin enough, we're not smart enough, we're not pretty enough or fit enough or educated or successful enough, or rich enough—ever. Before we even sit up in bed, before our feet touch the floor, we are already inadequate, already behind, already losing, already lacking something. And by the time we go to bed at night, our minds race with a litany of what we didn't get, didn't get done, that day. We go to sleep burdened by those thoughts and wake up to the reverie of lack. [...] What begins as a simple expression of the hurried life, or even the challenged life, grows into the great justification for an unfulfilled life.

An outgrowth of the scarcity thinking that Lynne Twist describes is comparison. You see, we measure our worth and our lack by comparing ourselves to someone else. In teaching the danger of comparison, Marshall Rosenberg, the creator of *Non-Violent Communications,* often asked his workshop participants to compare themselves to models on the magazine covers or successful famous people, who seemingly have accomplished a lot in their lives. If we tried that and compared ourselves to a model or an accomplished celebrity, how would we feel? Chances are, we would feel inadequate, unaccomplished, and small. Unfortunately, Instagram and other social media platforms perpetuate this violence by forcing near constant comparison between people who merely lead mundane existences and glamourous, beautiful influencers who always find themselves in exotic locations and always have clever, funny, and insightful things to say. Of course, if even 10% of people's actual lives resembled their Instagram posts we would be living in a very different world.

Scarcity thinking and endless comparisons lead to compulsive consumption—another critical way we express our violence. American Public Television's TV Show, *Affluenza* brought attention to the "epidemic of stress, overwork, waste, and indebtedness caused by the dogged pursuit of the American Dream." This, by the way, is not just limited to Americans, as overconsumption is a global phenomenon with wide ranging impacts on our entire planet and beyond. For example, if we just look at the consumption of red meat, now an expected daily staple around the world, it not only results in immeasurable cruelty to highly complex, clever, and social beings such as cows, lamb, and pigs, but also is one of the largest contributors to greenhouse emissions and thus the warming of the planet. In fact, the climate impact of red meat consumption is roughly equivalent to all the driving and flying of every car, truck, and plane in the world. The United Nations reported that the meat and dairy industries create 7.1 gigatons of greenhouse gasses annually—that's 14.5% of total man-made emissions.[37] Another way overconsumption of red meat contributes to climate change is via the destruction of forests and other habitats to make way for pasture. In pursuit of profits, ranchers are destroying hundreds of thousands of square miles of rainforest—vital, biodiverse ecosystems that, when undisturbed, capture millions of tons of CO_2. There is also an enormous impact on water as it takes on average about 15,415 liters of water to produce one kilo of beef. Moreover, manure lagoons used in livestock production—

which contain toxins and pathogens—present significant contamination risk for surface and ground waters.[38]

I use the example of meat just because it is something easily relatable to a large number of people. It would take several books and then some to detail all the ways in which our compulsive consumption negatively impacts both ourselves and the world. Of course, our compulsive consumption patterns include not just things and commodities, but also highly toxic information, which perpetuates highly charged and simplistic "victim/victor," and "us" vs. "them" narratives, desensitizes us to graphic violence and everyday cruelty, reinforce stereotypes, and even changes our sleeping and eating patterns. A co-worker once confided in me that she had difficulties falling asleep at night and did not feel rested in the morning. When I questioned her about her daily activity patterns, she revealed that upon waking up she would immediately check her phone for incoming emails. After getting up and making her first cup of coffee (she would need several more to get her going), she would turn on the local news. Local news outlets in America gleefully feed their viewers a steady diet of sensationalized and graphic stories of local crimes, gruesome car accidents, and over-dramatic weather reports. These are sprinkled with a few superficial national head-lines and one or two feel-good local stories. While on the train on her way to work, my co-worker passed the time by scrolling through her social media feeds. At work, she spent the entire day glued to her computer, while downing several energy drinks just to be able to stay awake. At night, following dinner with her partner, she watched *Law & Order SVU*. *Law & Order SVU* was a popular TV show for a number of years in America. SVU stands for Special Victims Unit—a major sex crime unit of the New York Police Department. The show graphicly depicted investigations and prosecutions of violent sex crimes in New York. My conversation with my colleague took place a number of years ago, before streaming platforms like Netflix, Amazon Prime, and Hulu gained in popularity. As graphic as *Law & Order SVU* was, it pales in comparison to even most benign shows on Amazon Prime or Netflix. Before going to bed, my colleague spent another hour or two scrolling through social media or surfing YouTube. I suspect that my co-worker's information consumption patterns are hardly out of the ordinary. Yet, is it really surprising that she had trouble sleeping?

Scarcity thinking, comparison, and compulsive consumption all stem from a fundamental confusion between what is *ours* and what is *us*. As we mistakenly believe that we are our accumulations, we continue to endlessly perpetuate this cycle of violence.

We could fill a library or two detailing all the ways we express our violence while showing unimaginable cruelty towards ourselves and other beings. In fact, in the next chapter we will talk about our propensity for judgements, evaluations, and conclusions—yet another way we express our violence. We may even be revisiting the "us" vs. "them" binary and exclusion when we talk about expansion.

One of the key critical reasons for tuning inward is to develop awareness of our innate (and as seen above, nearly endless) propensity for violence. Awareness is the difference between compulsive and conscious action and thus between *re-action* and *response.* As Psychiatrist Viktor Frankl reminded us, our ability to respond is in the space between a stimulus and an action which follows the stimulus. Tuning inward is how we develop and expand that space and ensure that the action is in fact a *response.*

Tuning inward is also how we expand our idea of ourselves. In his book, *Inner Engineering: A Yogi's Guide to Joy* and in many of his public discourses Sadhguru often shares the story of his enlightenment. He talks about riding his motorcycle up Chamundi Hill, a well-known gathering spot in Mysore City, in the southern Indian state of Karnataka. Sadhguru shares that he sat down at his favorite rock near the top of the hill in the middle of the day and closed his eyes. He opened his eyes hours later as the dark was descending over Mysore, unaware of the passage of time. Sadhguru's eyes welled with tears, and there was a profound change in the way that he was and the way he was experiencing everything and everyone around him. As he describes it, he could no longer tell where he ended and another being or even thing began. In experiencing everything and everyone as part of him, Sadhguru's life changed in the most profound of ways. In fact, this single experience is what transformed Jagi Vasudev, a businessman from Mysore City, into world-renown mystic, Yogi, and humanitarian we now know as Sadhguru.

Regardless of whether we reach the level of expansion of Sadhguru and other enlightened beings, tuning inward will naturally make us more inclusive, and thus less prone to violence. Just imagine how would we be if we experienced even for a moment the entirety of existence as part of us? This is not as wild as it may seem. Yes, each of us is a miniscule, micro-drop in the ocean of life. Yet, just as the ocean contains trillions of drops, every drop contains the ocean. I make no claims to enlightenment, yet in a very subtle way, expanding my idea of myself is what I experienced during my motorcycle journey through the Himalayas and my experience of expansion was a deep sense of inclusion. When our idea of ourselves expands we naturally become less rigid, more tolerant, and more inclusive. In my experience, inclusion is the most powerful antidote to violence. In fact, love is the ultimate act of inclusion. It expands our idea of ourselves in such a way where we include another being as part of *us,* seeing *their* wellbeing as being even more important than *ours.* Thus, the famous biblical quote— love thy neighbor—is a powerful teaching in inclusion.

Tuning inward is also how we start developing a distinction between what is *ours* and what *us.* Only by tuning inward can we realize our ultimate nature and end the endless cycle of separation, exclusion, contempt, scarcity, comparison, and over-consumption.

Tuning inward is also an important way to develop our connection to *this* moment. Life is not happening in our memory or in our imagination, as powerful and important as these faculties are in our experience. Rather, life is happening at this very moment, right here and right now. In fact, our experience in *this moment* touches on the very essence of life, being the only thing that is truly real. As Buddhist Monk and Scholar Thich Nhat Hanh put it: "The past no longer exists, and the future is not here yet." Ancient sage, Patanjali, began his *Yoga Sutras* with an easy to miss and infinitely profound half-sentence: "And, **Now** Yoga" (emphasis supplied). As Anand Mehrotra points out in his prolific commentary on the *Sutras*, *This is That*,

> Right at the outset Patanjali is declaring that yoga can only happen Now. Yoga can only be understood Now. Yoga can only be practiced Now. You can only experience yoga Now.

By connecting with the present moment, we are connecting with Yoga—not with the yoga of twisting and turning, but with Yoga—the practice, the experience, and the state of union with the creation and the creator, and thus with the very essence of life. Connection with the present moment is why the mantra: "I Am Here Now" is such an important part of the Dis-Solving Conflict from Within process.

Finally, tuning inward is how we tune into the very essence of life, as the source of all our experiences is within us. In *Inner Engineering: A Yogi's Guide to Joy* Sadhguru put it best:

> Everything that ever happened to you, you experienced right within you. Light and darkness, pain and pleasure, agony and ecstasy—all of it happened within you. If someone touches your hand right now, you may think you are experiencing their hand, but the fact of the matter is you are only experiencing the sensations in your own hand. The whole experience is contained within. All human experience is one hundred percent self-created.

The Experience of Tuning Inward

During one of my trips to India I stayed overnight in a small hotel in the ancient, holy city of Rishikesh. The hotel itself was pretty unremarkable but for the fact that the banks of the mighty Ganges River were just down a steep stairway from the main entrance to the hotel. On that particular day I woke up at five in the morning and felt the urge to go and spend some time with the Gangha Ma—the Mother Ganges, as the locals lovingly call the river. At five in the morning in early November the nearby Laxman Jhula Bridge which generally swelled with people, animals, and motorcycles, was empty but for a single cow. Gusting wind was playing a chilling game somewhere in the distance with two small metal objects. As I made my way down the steep stairwell to the beach of sorts, I saw the mist rising from the dark waters, which seemed more threatening than motherly. Shadows of animals, mostly street dogs and cows, though I could not tell in the dark, and people, likely Sadhus, were lurking in the background. The atmosphere was eerie, cold, and uninviting. I sat on the cold, damp ground and closed my eyes. And then, tears, seemingly endless waves of tears began to flow. I was weeping uncontrollably and inconsolably like I have never wept before. Deep sobs kept coming in overwhelming and consuming waves. To this day I have no idea why I cried. My tears on that day were not tears of sadness, neither, however, were they tears of joy. When I finally stopped, I had no idea how much time had elapsed, though it was light and the town was beginning to buzz with early morning life.

My experience by the Gangha was one of the clearest illustrations for me of what tuning inward is and isn't about. Starting with the latter, it isn't about thinking or analyzing—I don't recall having any thoughts as I sat by the Gangha. Nor is tuning inward about reaching some inner Nirvana where beautiful angels sing while being bathed in soft, white light. As I mentioned, while the tears poured out of me I was not particularly joyous. Finally, tuning inward is not about becoming obsessive about what we are experiencing.

What tuning inward *is* about being *willing* to *unconditionally* be with whatever is arising within us, whether what's arising is tears, or laughter, or anything in between. Being with something unconditionally means we don't try to fix or change it in any way. Ironically, when we sit with something unconditionally, fully willing to experience what is, the very nature of our experience changes. Naturally, some space starts to develop between our experience and us. In this space we are able to see the experience as something that is arising through us, but isn't us. When I cried by the Ganga, I was very aware of the sensations of crying—deep sobs that reverberated through my body; breath undulations, caused by waves of tears; and tears streaming down my cheeks. Yet, at the same time, somehow, I was removed from my experience. I was able to observe this being and feel immense compassion for him. While crying uncontrollably, inside I was at peace and at ease.

The Practice of Tuning Inward

One way to practice tuning inward is to incorporate the Dis-Solving Conflict from Within process into one's daily routine, whether one is going through conflict or not. Over time, the regular practice of the process creates more spaciousness within us. More spaciousness within us translates into more space between all of our accumulations and us, whether the accumulations are of the body, or of the mind. The more space there is between us and all of our accumulations, the more profound our very experience of life becomes, and the less impact everything that is outside of us, and especially conflict, has on us. And, because of the impact tuning inward could have on our life, the Dis-Solving Conflict from Within process could be an important step in tuning inward, but the process by itself is not enough.

One of the most critical tools for tuning inward is the regular practice of meditation. While meditation is becoming increasingly more mainstream in the West, I routinely encounter profound misunderstandings of meditation, even from people who claim to be "mindfulness" and/or "meditation" and/or "yoga" experts. In fact, many people complain to me that they are "not good at meditation" because their idea of meditation is that all of a sudden their brain activity should cease and they should experience no thought. Of course, applying this standard means that people who are clinically dead, or under heavy anesthesia, are enlightened meditation masters. Nor is meditation an occasional stress management or relaxation tool, or a quick escape to a more pleasant place.

In my experience, meditation is, first and foremost, absolute willingness to be with what is, even if what it means is that we not only experience the monkey mind, but we got a whole Planet of the Apes going on. As one Buddhist Master put it, sometimes the experience of meditation is touching Nirvana, and sometimes it's like putting our head up a dust bin. Second, meditation is a consistent practice which trains the mind to establish and maintain focus, without the tension we associate with it in the West. Ultimately, meditation is a state which effortlessly combines dynamism and stillness, focus and relaxation, alertness and withdrawal. It is the ultimate state of intensity but without the tension. It is the ability to be absolutely involved with life, but without getting entangled. Meditation is the practice, experience, and the state of observation without evaluation. It is awareness in its purest form and the ultimate connection with this moment and with the very essence of what life is and with who and what we are.

The practice of meditation has a few critical components to make it truly effective. Consistency is number one. When I was in India, I encountered many spiritual seekers who were in the business of collecting practices and Gurus. As a general rule, these folks had beautiful Instagram feeds, filled with meaningful sayings and pictures of themselves in various exotic locales. Yet, the new age façade was unstable. It seemed that the slightest provocation revealed cynicism, passive aggression, and escapism. Talking about the importance of consistency of meditation practice Anand Mehrotra put it best when he likened meditation practice to digging for water in the desert. Making small holes all over is unlikely to get one to water. On the other hand, digging consistently in one place just might. Consistency when it comes to meditation means picking one practice and sticking with it on a regular, preferably daily, basis over time.

Another critical component of meditation is to actually focus within. In recent years there has been a proliferation of various meditation apps. I think they can be helpful in getting one initially inspired to practice meditation. Some guided meditations, led by true masters, can be deep, transformative, and profound. However, with apps there is still focus outside of us—we need a phone, an app, someone's voice, and perhaps music to create a particular experience for us. While meditating with an app is better than not meditating at all, it is not the optimal experience as the focus is on the app and not within us.

The final critical component of meditation is patience. It takes time to develop a consistent practice and to start seeing some benefit from it. Initially, the mind will get bored and the body will become stiff. Five minutes will feel like excruciating hours. It will feel like you have more errant thoughts than you have ever had and you will be convinced that meditation is an impossible feat, perhaps accessible to Buddha and few other enlightened beings, but impenetrable to mere mortals.

That is exactly how I felt when I first learned Transcendental Meditation™ nearly fourteen years ago. Yet, I cannot think of another tool that has been more impactful on every aspect of my life. Before meditation became a part of my life, I was deeply insecure about myself, was constantly anxious, and fearful. During a typical day I was either jittery or lethargic, downing sugar and caffeine multiple times per day as pickups. I craved approval from other people and the slightest sign of disapproval made me fearful and worried. Maintaining consistent focus and concentration was a challenge. While I liked being a lawyer, I was almost in a constant state of overwhelm. I got things done, though my overall productivity was pretty low.

My personal relationships were up and down roller coasters. I married a woman whom I loved, though a few years into our marriage our relationship was on the rocks. Alas, there were not any major issues in our marriage, just the cumulative weight of many minor annoyances which made both of us question if we wanted to stay together. In fact, it was a marriage and family therapist we saw who first taught us meditation and suggested that we try to meditate as a tool for staying together. We didn't know if we would stay together or apart, but we hoped we would grow from the experience. Little did we know how meditation would change both of our lives.

Every day now I start my day with nearly a three-hour meditation and yoga practice. This is my daily anchor and an integral part of my life. In fact, just as it is hard for me to imagine leaving my home without having brushed my teeth, it is hard to imagine facing the world without having meditated. I credit my daily practice with transforming my life into a life of ease, inspiration, impact, abundance, connection, and expansion. I am happy to report that my relationship with Juliya morphed into a deeper, more intimate, and more meaningful connection. It's not that challenges have disappeared from my life, it's just that my capacity to deal with them has increased exponentially. The past year and a half crystalized how much I have changed. Over the past year and a half, I have incurred substantial business losses which were in part responsible for Juliya and I selling our comfortable home of ten years. Uncertainty over our next steps resulted in Juliya and I moving in with her parents. Then I got a job in Virginia, eight hours away from where my loved ones were, in an environment which was completely new to me. Because of Juliya's job and our living arrangements, every two weeks I commuted between Virginia and Pennsylvania. This was all right before Covid-19. As Covid hit, we curbed all of our social connections and delayed our move to Virginia. Then, in the spring of last year I fell from a bicycle and injured my knee. It turned out that I had torn both my ACL and my meniscus, and had to undergo knee reconstruction surgery followed by months of rehab. Also, my mom, a highly vulnerable individual from a health perspective, caught Covid (she has since recovered). Before meditation, every one of these events would have had a monumental impact on me and the combined effect of these would have been a tsunami. While I cannot say that these events did not impact me, what once would have been a tsunami is now a wave, and what once was a wave is now merely a ripple.

One of the easiest ways to practice meditation is to utilize breath. Breath is an ever-present life force that can not only connect us to the present moment but also enable us to traverse into higher layers of consciousness. The Connected Breathing Technique is in essence a very simple form of breath-based meditation practice. Another breathing technique that can be very helpful is called Alom Vilom breath. This technique is also known as alternate nostril breathing. This technique clears and balances left and right currents of the spine, and brings one into focused, but relaxed state of ease. To practice this technique we will use the pinky and thumb of the right hand to alternatively close the nostrils. While seated in a comfortable position with eyes closed, use the right thumb to close the right nostril, while inhaling through the left. Upon completing the inhale, remove the right thumb and use the pinky to close the left nostril and exhale through the right. Inhale through the right while closing the left nostril and then upon completing the inhale, close the right nostril with the right thumb and exhale through the left. I practice this technique before any meeting or interaction where I would like to be especially present and focused. Later on I will talk about how to incorporate this and other techniques I talk about in this chapter into a very powerful daily practice.

Another tool that is very helpful in meditation is part of both the transcendental and vedic traditions, and that's mantra. Mantra is a technology of using certain sounds to create particular experiences in the body. In Sanskrit "Man" means heart and "Tra" means expansion or liberation. In my experience, Sanskrit mantras are especially helpful in meditation as Sanskrit is a sacred language where many of the words were specifically designed to not only convey a particular meaning, but also to create a particular experience. In my daily meditation practice, I utilize a special Sanskrit mantra that my teacher has initiated me into, which I find to be both powerful and effective. I invite you to consider integrating mantra meditation into your practice utilizing a very simple Sanskrit mantra: Aham Brahmasmi, which translates as "I am totality, totality is me." To practice this mantra-meditation, sit in a comfortable seated position with spine comfortably erect and away from any backing. Close your eyes. As you inhale, think of the word "Aham". As you exhale, think of the word "Brahmasmi." If any thoughts or sensations come, return to the phrase. As you sit and practice, the phrase may move to the background and eventually even disappear. Don't try to bring the phrase back if it does not naturally come, but just sit with whatever is.

A word about meditation apps. People I work with often proudly share with me that they have a daily meditation practice where they use various meditation apps, like Headspace or InsightTimer, to tune in. In my experience, these meditation apps offer wonderful relaxation techniques. Relaxation techniques are wonderful, but they are very different from meditation. As we discussed, the purpose of meditation is not to relax (it can be a very nice side effect), but to learn to unconditionally be with whatever *is* in the moment. For that, I find breath and mantra based meditations that do not depend on access to a phone or wi-fi to be most effective.

Another important aspect of tuning inward for me has been a daily practice of kriyas. Kriyas are an ancient yogic technology of personal transformation. Known as evolutionary action, Kriyas combine particular patterns of breath, mantras, and/or movement to impact and transform subtler dimensions of human experience. I first was exposed to kriyas while practicing Sattva Yoga in India, and was astonished by how powerfully transformative kriyas were. Sattva Yoga, which translates as "holistic" yoga, is a series of practices developed and taught by Anand Mehrotra. To understand how kriyas work, we need to touch on yogic understanding of the human body. In the yoga tradition the human body is seen as consisting of five koshas. Kosha means layer or sheath. In looking at Koshas we go from the grossest, or the most perceptible by the senses, to the subtlest, or the least visible to us. The first layer or sheath is Annamaya Kosha, or the food body. This is the most physical dimension of the body and consists of limbs, tissue, organs, and fluids that make up the physical body. The second layer is called Pranamaya Kosha. Prana means energy. Pranamaya Kosha represents the energy that flows and animates matter, bringing it to life. In other words, Pranamaya Kosha is like electricity which flows from the light switch to the light bulb, making the light bulb glow. The third layer of the body is called Manomaya Kosha. *Mano* is the closest Sanskrit word to the English word *mind*. So, Manomaya Kosha is the mind layer of the body. The Yogic idea of the mind is much more expansive than the Western one, as yogis never saw the mind as being limited to the brain only. Rather, Manomaya Kosha is present in all parts of the body and includes conscious and unconscious memory, intellect, intelligence, emotions, and what we would call individuality. Manomaya Kosha also includes the human capacities for self-awareness, connection, and higher-level thinking. Annamaya, Pranamaya, and Manomaya Koshas are all physical, it's just that Pranamaya and Manomaya Koshas are more subtle than the Annamaya Kosha. Vigyanamaya Kosha, the fourth layer, is the link between physical and non-physical aspects of existence. As the word *Vigyana* means knowledge, it is associated with higher-level knowledge, which goes beyond the intellect. It is probably best described as the experience of two higher and non-physical dimensions of our existence—*Sat*, the ultimate, the absolute truth of who we are, and *Chit*, consciousness the unity of all existence. The final Kosha is called Anandamaya Kosha—the bliss layer. This layer is purely non-physical and non-local to the body and refers to the unity between creator and creation. There is no description for this layer as yogis believed it to be beyond the comprehension of the human mind. Though, when one touches this layer of existence, they experience pure and unbound bliss.

Kriyas are practices specifically designed to impact Pranamaya, Manomaya, and even Vijnanamaya Koshas. In other words, Kriyas work on and with the body's subtle energies and even touch on non-physical and mystical aspects of existence. Because Kriyas are such powerful tools of transformation, they require advanced knowledge and very special care. That is why traditionally kriyas were passed through the generations by the Gurus to their disciples. In modern times, however, kriyas are much more accessible. The two kriya-based practices I have personal experience with are taught by Sadhguru and by Anand Mehrotra. Sadhguru offers two kriya-based yoga programs—base-level *Inner Engineering* and the more advanced *Shoonya Program*. Information about Sadhguru's programs is available at: www.innerengineering.com. Sattva Yoga kriya-based practices, specifically including practices personally taught by Anand Mehrotra are available at: www.sattvaconnect.com. Just to illustrate how powerful kriya practices are, I am going to share a kriya practice below called Sudarshan Kriya III. I learned this kriya in India from Anand Mehrotra. It is part of the Sattva Yoga practice.

Sudarshan Kriya III increases overall vitality, releases stress and toxins, improves the immune system, creates a sense of clarity, commitment and purpose. This kriya is very helpful when going through any tense or stressful experience and especially so when going through conflict. It should be practiced on an empty stomach, preferably in the morning. To practice this kriya sit in a cross-legged posture, placing the left heel under the perineum (the area between the anus and the sexual organ) with right leg being in front of the left leg. Keep the spine comfortably erect and close your eyes. Inhale deeply and close the right nostril with the right thumb and exhale through the left nostril. While holding the breath out, pump the stomach without moving the breath 7, 14, or 21 times. Inhale deeply through the left nostril. Close the left nostril with the right pinky upon completing the inhale and exhale through the right nostril. Inhale through the right nostril. Hold the breath in and pump the stomach without moving the breath 7, 14, or 21 times. Exhale through the right nostril then inhale through the right nostril and then exhale through the right nostril. Hold the breath out and pump the stomach without moving the breath for 7,14 or 21 times. After pumping, inhale through the right nostril and while closing the right nostril with your thumb, exhale from the left. Inhale from the left nostril and while holding the breath in, pump the stomach 7, 14, or 21 times. Exhale from the left nostril, inhale from the left nostril and exhale from the left nostril. Pump the stomach without breathing 7, 14, or 21 times. This is one complete cycle of the Sudarshan Kriya. Practice this kriya for 5–7 minutes. It is important to pump the stomach a consistent number of times both while holding the breath in and holding the breath out. So, if you pump 14 times while holding the breath out, be sure to pump 14 times while holding the breath in. Women who are menstruating can still practice this Kriya, but should not use full-force pumps. Women who are pregnant should avoid this kriya. Note, it is not unusual to experience some light-headedness or light headache after practicing this kriya. If this occurs, sit quietly, while focusing on your breath practicing the Connected Breathing Technique until symptoms dissipate. Additional instructions along with video demonstration and audio guidance for practicing this kriya are available at: www.livingpeaceinstitute.com.

While meditation and kriya yoga are very important aspects of tuning inward, some additional aspects should not be overlooked. Tuning inward also includes developing general awareness of what we contribute to the world. This is one place where I think binary choice is appropriate. Either through our actions, our consumption, and our general presence we are contributing to peace, harmony, connection, and inclusion in the world, or we are contributing to division, contempt, and lack. This is not about judging, but rather about cultivating awareness so that as many of our actions as possible become conscious actions, rather than compulsive ones. Tuning inward also includes communion with nature; journaling; maintaining and developing conscious and nurturing connections; self-care; regular laughter; preferably a vegetarian diet, rich in simple foods which grow; and overall commitment to living from within.

Another important aspect of tuning inward is the practice of devotion. Devotion is not about a belief in a particular deity, whatever name we may give it. Rather, Devotion is an intentional cultivation of gratitude, trust, humility, and equanimity accessible to us irrespective of circumstances we might find ourselves in. Devotion is about enlivening the space and moment where we are and being in the state of absolute receptivity. It is a deep longing to realize our ultimate nature and to discover the distinction between what is *ours* and what is *us*. Devotion begins with full and unconditional acceptance of this moment. As Sadhguru teaches in one of his most profound teachings, "this moment is just the way it is. It can't be any other way." This is the very essence of the Yogic teaching of Santosha or equanimity. As Anand Mehrotra describes in his commentary on the *Yoga Sutras* by Patanjali:

> This practice of equanimity is the dropping of all resistance to what is, the letting go of this whole story about what you have, what you don't have, who you are, what you would rather be and chasm in between filled with conflict. As you allow this equanimity to rise, you start to acknowledge the bit that is your life in every breath you take. A deep state of appreciation in what is then starts to rise and in that state of appreciation, you are naturally filled with energy [and] vitality[39].

When we accept this moment just the way it is, we dis-solve one of the most enduring conflicts—the conflict between presence or what is and *us*.

Thus, the practice of the Dis-Solving Conflict from Within process, and especially the mantra, "I" "am" "here" "now" is itself a powerful tool of devotion. Other ways to bring devotion into our lives include enlivening the spaces where we are at. Something as simple as lighting a candle or an oil lamp, bringing flowers and fresh water into the space where we are at and simply bowing down to the great mystery, the great unknown that is this life, can shift our inner state in the most powerful and profound ways. When I lived in India, we began each day with a special Bhuta Shuddhi Puja or a ceremony honoring and awakening all the elements. This was a simple process involving singing of mantras, lighting an oil lamp, and making an offering of water, flowers, and fruit. Somehow this ceremony brought a different dimension to my experience. Whenever I partook in this ceremony, it was as though someone removed a thin veil from my face, bringing greater vibrancy, richness, and sensitivity to my experience of life. While we only occasionally do this ceremony at home, I always finish my daily practice with a bow to life. In my experience it has made a difference.

Suggested Daily Practice

For us to truly experience the transformative impacts of tuning inward so that tuning inward becomes our normal state, practice is a must. Below is the proposed daily practice regiment which incorporates the techniques we discussed above as well as the Dis-Solving Conflict from Within process. Please, commit to this practice daily for a period of 40 days.

Wake up and light an oil lamp, and perhaps bring some fresh flowers to enliven your space

Alom Vilom Breath (5–10 minutes)

Dis-Solving Conflict from Within Process (10 minutes or 2 complete rounds)

Sudarshan Kriya III (7–10 minutes)

Aham Brahmasmi Meditation (15–30 minutes)

Bow to life while bringing your forehead to the ground

Before Going to Sleep:

Alom Vilom Breath (5 minutes)

Gratitude Practice (Tuning in to all the things you are grateful for. Do this especially if you are transitioning through challenges).

If you commit to the above practice on a daily basis for a period of at least 40 days, I guarantee you that your conflict interactions will be transformed. Your conflict interactions will be transformed because you will be showing up to your conflict interactions and to your life as a different—more aware, less violent, and more inclusive—person.

8

OBSERVATION
WITHOUT EVALUATION

"What's wrong with you!!!"
"What an idiot!!!"
"She has such a big mouth!!!"
"I am a failure!!!"
"He always gets it wrong!"
"My teammates are just not collaborative!"

Perhaps you have heard some variation of the above phrases and perhaps even used such phrases yourself. If we are honest, just about everything we say is some sort of a judgment, evaluation, label, or conclusion. This is especially true of our inner dialogue. And I don't think Twitter would be around for long without these. Judgements, evaluations, labels, and conclusions are yet another way we stay in our violence. What makes these so dangerous is that they are precursors to shame, both our own and weaponized towards others. In her best-selling book, *The Gifts of Imperfection: Let Go of Who You Think You're Supposed To Be and Embrace Who You Are*, Brené Brown defines shame as the intensely painful experience of believing that we are so flawed that we are unworthy of love and belonging. She continues:

> ...[i]t is human nature to want to feel worthy of love and belonging. When we experience shame, we feel disconnected and desperate for worthiness. Full of shame or the fear of shame, we are more likely to engage in self-destructive behaviors and to attack or shame others. In fact, shame is related to violence, aggression, depression, addiction, eating disorders, and bullying.

The antidote to judgements, labels, evaluations, and conclusions are observations. The key distinction between observations and judgments, labels, evaluations, and conclusions is that observations focus on the behavior rather than the person. Thus, observations allow for guilt (i.e. I did something bad), but banish shame (i.e. I am bad). So critical is the skill of observation without evaluation, judgment, label, or conclusion, that the 20th Century Indian philosopher, Jiddhu Krishnamurti, called it the highest form of intelligence. Likewise, Sadhguru referred to the ability to listen as "the essence of intelligent living." However, it is singer/songwriter and student of Non-Violent Communications, Ruth Bebermeyer who truly captured the essence of observation without evaluation in her song/poem:

> *I've never seen a lazy man;*
> *I've seen a man who never ran*
> *while I watched him, and I've seen*
> *a man who sometimes slept between*
> *lunch and dinner, and who'd stay*
> *at home upon a rainy day, but he was not a lazy man.*
> *Before you call me crazy,*
> *Think, was he a lazy man or*
> *did he just do things we label "lazy"?*

I've never seen a stupid kid;
I've seen a kid who sometimes did
things I didn't understand
or things in ways I hadn't planned;
I've seen a kid who hadn't seen
the same places where I had been,
but he was not a stupid kid.
Before you call him stupid,
think, was he a stupid kid or did he
just know different things that you did?

I've looked as hard as I can look
but never ever seen a cook;
I saw a person who combined
ingredients on which we dined,
A person who turned on the heat
and watched the stove that cooked the meat—
I saw those things but not a cook.
Tell me, when you're looking,
Is it a cook you see or is it someone
doing things that we call cooking?

What some of us call lazy
some call tired or easy-going,
what some call stupid
some just call a different knowing
so, I've come to the conclusion,
it will save us all confusion
if we don't mix up what we can see
with what is our opinion.
Because you may, I want to say also;
I know that's only my opinion.

To start practicing this highest form of intelligence, we first must develop awareness of when we judge, label, evaluate or conclude and then consciously switch to an observation. Some examples are below:

- Susan's got a big mouth! (judgment, evaluation)
- Susan shared information I've asked her not to share. (observation)
- John is disrespectful! (label)
- During our last meeting John interrupted me three times. (observation)
- Terri is racist! (label, judgment, and conclusion)
- In her comment on Twitter, Terri used language I found to be offensive. (observation)
- Sam will forget to do what I've asked him. He always does! (conclusion)
- I don't know if Sam will remember to do what I've asked. In the past, there were times when they forgot. (observation)

I invite you to start noticing (of course, without judging yourself!) when you label, judge, or evaluate and then consciously switch to an observation. This is something that will powerfully transform all of your interactions, including your interactions with yourself and with those you are having a conflict with.

Compassion in Action

One of the most powerful and effective ways to practice observation without evaluation is through the practice of active listening. I know active listening can be cliché, yet it is by far the most important and the most transformative tool I use every day in my work as a mediator, facilitator, coach, and teacher. I see active listening as compassion in action. Thus, it is one of the most potent ways to cultivate connection, transform conflict, and even respond to bullying and prejudice.

Since I brought up the "c" word—Compassion, I'd like to talk about compassion before we actually learn the skill of active listening. To understand compassion, we first need to understand pity, sympathy, and empathy.

Pity and sympathy both contain a mixture of inequality and judgment. The difference between these two is just in the degree of inequality and judgment they contain. To borrow an example from Brené Brown, suppose I fell into a deep hole and was in a very dark place, all alone. If you come by, look down the hole and exclaim: "I see you're in the hole. What a dumb and stupid thing to do. I would never do that! I feel bad for you!" You would be expressing pity. In the same situation if you come by, look down my hole and say: "I see you're in the hole. I feel bad for you. Maybe next time you should bring a ladder. And, at least this hole is not so deep." You would be expressing sympathy for me.

Empathy is where you would actually try to connect with my experience—try to feel what I'm feeling. Back to the dark, lonely hole I'm occupying. If you'd come by and say: "Wow, you're in the hole! I've been there myself. I know how you are feeling. Perhaps, let me climb down there with you so that we can stay together." You are expressing empathy for me. "Me Too!" could be a powerful and validating statement of comradery. This expression is also quite misleading, as even the same experiences could feel very differently to different people. And, what if we do not share an experience, or your experience is so painful, powerful and/or extraordinary that I could never even imagine how it would feel? This really came home for me when I was working with a father whose fifteen-year-old son committed suicide. I don't have children. How could I pretend that I know how this man felt? How could I even imagine being in his shoes even for a moment? Would it be insulting to this man's unimaginable pain and grief for me to even try?

If in empathy you try to feel what I'm feeling, in compassion you know you can't. Because even if you've been in the hole yourself, my experience of being in a hole could be completely different from yours. So, if I'm in a hole, in compassion you'd come by and say: "It looks like you are in a hole. I've been in many holes myself. Tell me, how are you feeling? What would be the most helpful thing I could do for you now? How could I serve?" Then, you would stay with me, listening fully and unconditionally to me, and thus empowering me to get out of the hole myself. As Canadian Buddhist nun, teacher, and author Pema Chödrön pointed out in her book, *Places that Scare You: A Guide to Fearlessness in Difficult Times*:

> Compassion is not a relationship between the healer and the wounded. It's a relationship between equals. Only when we know our own darkness well can we be present with the darkness of others. Compassion becomes real when we recognize our shared humanity.

So, compassion is knowing fully that we can never be in another person's shoes, but that by virtue of intimately knowing our own pain, we know the pain of being human and thus can unconditionally hold space for them. As we start learning the skill of active listening, let us treat it as a way to bring compassion to the world.

Active Listening

While many talk about active listening, few actually know how to do it and especially how to do it well. Active listening is the process of connecting with another human being by engaging fully and unconditionally with what they are saying. The purpose of active listening is understanding. There are four key aspects to active listening: preparing our body for listening; becoming aware of the times when we wish to interrupt the speaker; tuning-in to the e-motion, energy, and intensity behind the speaker's words; and reflecting back to the speaker the general gist of what they said, while capturing key e-motions and matching the speaker's intensity.

If you've ever gone running, probably before running you've put on your sneakers and performed some leg stretches. These simple acts prepare the body for running. Just like preparing the body for running, we need to take steps to prepare the body for listening. When ancient yogis wanted to enter deep states of meditation or when they were listening to their Master, the yogis would fold their tongue in such a way where the tip of the tongue would touch the soft spot behind the upper palette. This technique is called Kechari Mudra. If you could take a moment and fold your tongue just so and then try to say your name out loud. If you are having difficulty, you are experiencing the fact that this simple technique closes off your speaking channel, while opening the listening one. I use this technique all the time when I'm listening to other people or even when I'm riding motorcycles—these are the times when I would like to be the most attentive. Next, it would be very useful to sit with your spine tall and chest open. It is best to avoid folding our arms. We fold our arms when we try to prevent the outside from entering us. Thus, if the room you're sitting in all of a sudden got chilly, you would naturally fold your arms to prevent the chill from impacting you. It is also very helpful to focus on your breath as you listen. Maintaining deep, consistent breathing ensures that your brain is getting the oxygen it needs. An oxygenated, relaxed brain is also an attentive one. Finally, as you listen, use your body to communicate to the speaker that you are with them. Strong, uninterrupted eye contact, slight nods of the head, and attentive posture communicate to the speaker that you are with them. I avoid taking notes when listening so as to not break eye contact with the speaker.

As you listen to the speaker, there may be inclinations to jump in—to share how your situation might be similar to that of the speaker; to ask clarifying questions; to offer advice or solutions; or to inform the speaker that you know how they feel. It is best to avoid these interruptions as they interfere with the speaker's flow. As you start practicing active listening, I invite you to notice when you would like to jump in, and if possible, to resist this temptation.

When you listen, it is important to hear the speaker's words. However, it is also vital to tune in to the energy, intensity, and e-motion behind the words. Don't miss the vital while focusing on the important. It is the focus on the vital that will enable you not just to listen, but to actually hear and understand.

The final aspect of active listening, the aspect that is often missed, is reflection. Reflection is not about mindlessly mirroring the words of the speaker. Rather it is about capturing emotion and meaning behind the words. Here, don't be afraid to match the speaker's intensity. The more closely you can match the speaker's intensity, the more likely they will feel heard. And don't be afraid to get it wrong. The speaker will correct you and will appreciate your attempt to listen, hear, and understand.

I know practicing active listening can feel a bit awkward, especially when you do it with loved ones or close friends. I invite you to practice anyway, as active listening is the most direct pathway for radically transforming even the most challenging interactions into opportunities for understanding, connection, and inclusion.

In his June 26th, 2021 column, titled *How Can You Hate Me When You Don't Even Know Me?*, influential *New York Times* columnist Nicholas Kristof shared a powerful example of active listening in action. In his column, Kristof talked about Daryl Davis. Daryl Davis is a Black musician who chooses to spend his time with Ku Klux Klan members and neo-Nazis. Over the years, he has persuaded hundreds to leave hate behind. As Kristof writes:

> One of Davis' methods—there is research from social psychology to confirm the effectiveness of this approach—is not to confront antagonists and denounce their bigotry but rather to start in listening mode. Once people feel they are being listened to, [Davis] says, it is easier to plant a seed of doubt.

A former grand dragon of the Klan, Scott Shepherd, credits Davis with saving his life and empowering him to hang his robe and leave the life of hate behind. "Daryl extended his hand and actually just extended his heart, too, and we became brothers," said Shepherd. Daryl Davis' work with the Klan and neo-Nazis is well documented. In fact, I highly recommend Davis' TED talk and his podcast, *Changing Minds with Darryl Davis*. If listening could persuade hardened Klan members and neo-Nazis to leave hate behind, just think of how listening could transform our everyday conflicts!

While I use active listening many times a day and see its transformative power nearly every time I use it, I discovered the true power of it when training a group of police officers. This particular group of officers had to be at this training and they went out of their way to make it clear to me how much they resented it. Clearly, everyone was taking their clue from the gruff sergeant who sat in the back of the room with his arms folded and eyebrows frowned. Occasionally, and generally right in the midst of an important point or during my meager attempts at humor, the sergeant yawned loudly to remind everyone how little he thought of the whole spectacle and would have much rather been somewhere, anywhere else. This was a multi-day training and it clearly was not going well! After teaching active listening to the officers and giving them an assignment to practice it with their loved ones and friends, I secretly contemplated faking an illness so that I wouldn't have to show up the next day. I showed up the next day and continued the training. This time, my friend, a sergeant, sat in the front of the room. He was engaged, focused, and attentive. During one of the breaks in the training I approached him, joking that perhaps there was something wrong with the water in the building which caused such a change. The sergeant did not laugh but met my gaze and spoke. "Henry!" he addressed me. "Yesterday, when we started this training, I thought all of this was a bunch of bullshit!" the sergeant continued. "After all, you haven't spent a damn day on the street! So, what could you teach us?!" he added, followed by a pause that seemed way too long. "But, then you gave us this homework assignment—to try active listening. I still thought it was bullshit, but I decided to try it with my daughter," toughness melting away as the daughter came up. Now, it was time for me to be even more surprised as the sergeant's eyes welled with tears "You know, my daughter is an interesting person. I think this was the first time I actually listened to her, instead of just bossing her around. She has so much to say." The sergeant delivered the punchline while now slouching in his chair. With gruffness returning, the sergeant concluded: "Maybe, you're onto something here!"

9

EXPANSION

If there was ever a man with a legitimate grievance, Nelson Mandela was it. Since the time he was a young lawyer in Transvaal, he had spent years leading the struggle against Apartheid in South Africa. The personal toll the struggle took, which Mandela detailed in his brilliant autobiography *Long Walk to Freedom*, seems both unimaginable and unbearable. This toll included: spending years living in hiding; multiple betrayals; arrests; at least two show trials; the end of two marriages; and a twenty-nine year imprisonment. Mandela spent eighteen years of his confinement at Robben Island where he endured hard, back-breaking labor and abuse from white prison guards. While at Robben Island, Mandela also initiated several hunger strikes, protesting the treatment of Black prisoners. Bowing to international pressure and responding to increasing domestic unrest, South-African President F.W. de Klerk finally released Nelson Mandela from prison in 1990. Upon being released from prison, Mandela described his interaction with one of his jailers, a white Afrikaans man named James Gregory:

Warrant Officer James Gregory was also there at the house, and I embraced him warmly. In the years that he had looked after me from Pollsmoor through Victor Verster, we had never discussed politics, but our bond was an unspoken one and I would miss his soothing presence.

F.W. de Klerk came up through the ranks of the Nationalist Party, the very political movement of minority, white, Afrikaans South Africans responsible for apartheid—the years-long system of oppression and discrimination of Black South Africans and South Africans of Indian origin. Thus, de Klerk's act of releasing Mandela was more of an act of pragmatic survival rather than principled courage. In the years that followed as de Klerk and Mandela negotiated the end of Apartheid, de Klerk's obstruction was more than a bit frustrating to Mandela and his African National Congress colleagues.

Nonetheless, during a 1994 televised debate between Mandela and de Klerk as both were competing for the presidency of South Africa, Mandela said the following:

> The exchange between Mr. de Klerk and me should not obscure one important fact. I think we are a shining example to the entire world of people drawn from different racial groups who have a common loyalty, a common love, to their common country....We are going to face the problem of this country together...I am proud to hold your hand for us to go forward.

Later on when sharing the Nobel Peace Prize with de Klerk, Mandela honored de Klerk in his acceptance speech in Norway stating about de Klerk:

> He had the courage to admit that a terrible wrong had been done to our country and people through the imposition of the system of apartheid. He had the foresight to understand and accept that all the people of South Africa must, through negotiations and as equal

participants in the process, together determine what they want to make of their future.

Finally, when being inaugurated as South Africa's first black president, Mandela said the following:

> We thank all of our distinguished international guests for having come to take possession with the people of our country of what is, after all, a common victory for justice, for peace, for human dignity.
>
> We have, at last, achieved our political emancipation. We pledge ourselves to liberate all people from the continuing bondage of poverty, deprivation, suffering, gender, and other discrimination.

By the way, guests at Mandela's inauguration, specifically invited by him, included his former jailer, a prosecutor who sought the death penalty for Mandela, and one of the former leaders of apartheid in South Africa.

Mandela's sentiments included more than words. As President of South Africa, he focused on reconciliation between Black and White South Africans, encouraging Black South Africans to cheer for the previously much hated South African National Rugby Team and authorizing the creation of the National Truth and Reconciliation Commission, headed by another Nobel Laureate, Bishop Desmond Tutu.

Nelson Mandela was hardly a naïve person. He had no illusions about his jailers, F.W. de Klerk, and the complicity of white South Africans in the years of oppression he and his people endured. Yet, Mandela also understood the immense, transformative power of expansion and inclusion. Thus, Mandela chose to see humanity in his jailer and his political rival. He also understood that to build a new South Africa, he needed to expand beyond binary racial identities which for generations divided people to the broader and more inclusive identity of South Africans, engaged in building a new future for all of the country's citizens.

Another incredible being, who was one of Mandela's key inspirations, also understood the power of expansion. In his famous I Have a Dream speech, Dr. Martin Luther King, Jr. invoked the same themes of expansion and inclusion that Nelson Mandela would in his inaugural address over forty years later. On the steps of Washington Monument, Dr. King said in part:

Let us not wallow in the valley of despair, I say to you today, my friends.

And so even though we face the difficulties of today and tomorrow, I still have a dream. It is a dream deeply rooted in the American dream.

I have a dream that one day this nation will rise up and live out the true meaning of its creed: "We hold these truths to be self-evident, that all men are created equal."

I have a dream that one day on the red hills of Georgia, the sons of former slaves and the sons of former slave owners will be able to sit down together at the table of brotherhood.

I have a dream that one day even the state of Mississippi, a state sweltering with the heat of injustice, sweltering with the heat of oppression, will be transformed into an oasis of freedom and justice.

I have a dream that my four little children will one day live in a nation where they will not be judged by the color of their skin but by the content of their character.

Earlier in his life, King wrote from a Birmingham, Alabama jail:

In a real sense all life is inter-related. All men are caught in an inescapable network of mutuality, tied in a single garment of destiny. Whatever affects one directly, affects all indirectly. I can never be what I ought to be until you are what you ought to be, and you can never be what you ought to be, until I am what I ought to be.

From Positions to Needs

Actually, the way Mandela and King acted when faced with incredible adversity is anything but natural. In fact, it is much more natural for us to shrink and constrict. When in conflict, we enter a warp of sorts where we narrowly focus on past grievances and future anxieties, seeing those who trigger us as grotesque, dehumanized caricatures out to get us. Escaping this warp takes conscious and very deliberate movement from positions to needs.

In their well-known book, *Getting to Yes: Negotiating Agreement Without Giving In*, co-founders of the Harvard Negotiation Project Roger Fisher and William Ury used a poignant example to illustrate the need to move beyond positions in negotiations. Fisher and Ury used an example of two children arguing over an orange. A slightly dramatized version of this conversation is below:

"I want the orange," yelled one child.

"No, I want one," loudly shrieked the other one.

The children escalated by restating each of their respective desires for an orange by increasing their volume and intensifying their attitude.

"Enough!!!" exclaimed the children's father, walking from another room Thi. "Give me the knife!" As the father was about to cut the orange in half to put an end to the screaming, hearing all the commotion, the mom walked in. "Hang on a moment," she told the father and turned to the kids. "Why do you need the orange?" mom asked the first child. "I want the rinds to bake the scones." they exclaimed. The mom then turned to the second child "what about you, why do you want the orange?" "I want pulp to make juice" the child yelled in between sobs. So, here was the perfect solution—by asking one simple question the mom went beyond the children's position and identified their interests. Both children could get exactly what they wanted, without having to give up anything of value to either of them.

The above example is neat—it uses a simple and relatable situation and makes a very clear point. In my experience, this example is also incomplete and somewhat misleading. In my work with many conflicting parties, I have yet to come across someone who is that clear about their interests, and I have yet to see two siblings whose relationship is so straightforward where a simple, transactional solution truly satisfies everyone's interests. I've also discovered that to truly transform conflict, looking at interests is not enough. There are several more critical layers we need to explore to get at what is truly behind the conflict.

When teaching students and talking about expansion in the context of conflict transformation, I often use an analogy of an iceberg.

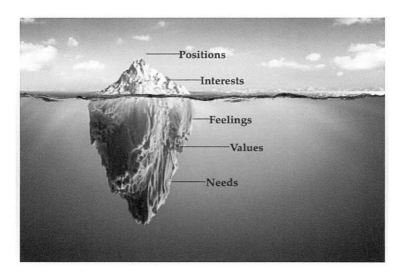

At the very tip of the iceberg are positions. Being at the tip, positions are the most superficial and thus least revealing layer of conflict. Unfortunately, despite this layer being the most superficial, that is where most conflicts stay. Certainly, when I practiced law, very few conflicts and even fewer attorneys went beyond purely positional arguments and transactional resolutions. Positional conflicts are also what we mostly see in our political discourse. Name calling prevalent on social media and slogans which pass for policy proposals on Twitter are great examples of positional arguments.

Right below positions, though still above the water level, are interests. In essence, interests are the reasons we hold particular positions. In my experience, people hold their positions for all kinds of irrational and even violent reasons. For instance, someone may express a particular position because it is a position expressed by the group the person feels affinity to; someone else may hold a position because they think this position will get them the result they want. While going beyond positions and thus deeper, the interest level is still relatively superficial. It is definitely not yet a place to stop. Digging deeper and expanding further is a must!

The next layer, which I picture right at the water level of the iceberg, are e-motions. If we are really interested in truly understanding someone, we must connect with the energies moving through them. This is why the practice of active listening is so critical—it enables us to hear and connect with the e-motions of the people we are listening to. Once we start connecting with e-motions, we are beginning to get to some depth. As we will be learning later, in the chapter on Non-Violent Communications, e-motions are very important as they serve as messengers for our needs.

Now we are underwater and are really expanding. While we still have not reached the full depth, we are getting close. This is where we come to values. In his instrumental book *The 7 Habits of Highly Effective People*, Steven R. Covey compared our values to a compass. He wrote:

> Our struggle to put first things first can be characterized by the contrast between two powerful tools that direct us: the clock and the compass. The clock represents our commitments, appointments, schedules, goals, activities—what we do with, and how we manage our time. The compass represents our vision, values, principles, mission, conscience, direction—what we feel is important and how we lead our lives.

I echo what Covey said and would add that I see values as what we ultimately see as being the most important for us. Of course, our values are influenced by culture, conditioning, and social situations. Yet, if we really dig deep into what is important to us, we will find that there is a lot more commonality in our values, even among seemingly very different people. Values and principles take us deep. Still, they are not the last level of expansion.

As I see it, the last level of expansion in conflict is our needs. Our positions and interests may be all over the place. In very intense conflicts there might be some similarities between our e-motions. There is definitely going to be some commonality among most deeply held values. However, no matter who we are or where we come from, our fundamental needs are going to be the same. I know when talking about needs, many would have an immediate association with Maslow's needs hierarchy. I don't think of needs in terms of a hierarchy, but rather see them as psycho-physical energies of the body. Thus, I associate our needs with the Yogic system of the chakras. Chakras are vortexes of energy located throughout the body which represent different aspects of existence. While the purpose of Yoga and meditation is to move the energies from the grosser aspects to the subtler, or from lower chakras to the higher ones, all dimensions of existence have relevance in different settings and at different times. I believe connecting our needs to the chakras offers a more nuanced approach to understanding needs than a hierarchy. The basic representation of the seven core needs is below. We will go through them moving from the grosser to the subtler, and thus will start at the bottom of the below diagram.

Our first need is security. I associate this need with the root chakra, located at the very base of the spine and known in Sanskrit as Muladhara. The qualities of the Muladhara chakra are security and stability. When in disbalance, this chakra is associated with feelings of fear and disconnection.

The need for security includes the security of the body and thus whatever it takes (i.e. food, water, shelter, and basic safety) to keep the body alive. The need for security also includes stability or knowing the basic rules of how the world operates.

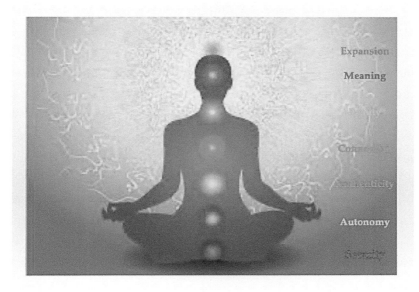

The second need is the need for autonomy, associated with the Swadisthana chakra. Physically, the Swadisthana chakra is below the belly button, right near the sex organ. The qualities of the Swadhisthana chakra include pleasure, desire, sexuality, and creativity. When in disbalance, Swadisthana becomes the center of addiction and identification with possessions (i.e. power, money, various accumulations, including the accumulation of knowledge).

The need for autonomy is fundamentally the need for self-determination—having a say in how we show up to life, what we desire, and how others perceive us.

I associate the third chakra called Manipura with the need for authenticity. Manipura, located in the navel center, is associated with personal power, dynamic action, assertiveness, and discipline. Manipura is also the maintenance center of the body. The need for authenticity translates to showing up to life from a place of strength, clarity about who we are (and what we are not), and ease. Of course, when we don't show up to life in an authentic way or someone is being inauthentic to us, it feels like a punch in the gut—hence another connection to the navel.

Anahata, or the heart chakra, is associated with a powerful and uniform need for connection. Our need for connection includes things like belonging, appreciation, and love. Brené Brown expressed the manifestation of this need in a way I found to be both relevant and powerful. In *Rising Strong: How the Ability to Reset Transforms the Way We Lead, Love, Parent, and Live* she wrote:

> Love will never be certain, but after collecting thousands of stories, I'm willing to call this a fact: A deep sense of love and belonging is an irreducible need of all men, women, and children. We are biologically, cognitively, physically, and spiritually wired to love, to be loved, and to belong.

I associate the fifth need, the need for beauty, with Vishuddha or the throat chakra. In the Yoga tradition, this chakra is associated with purification, transmutation, alchemy, and infinity. To me, all of these are associated with beauty, both natural and human-made. A beautiful piece of music or art, or a beautiful natural landscape has the power to purify us and is a reminder of the alchemy and infinity of life.

The need for meaning is connected with the Agya chakra, located in the middle of the forehead. In the Yoga tradition this chakra is associated with wisdom, intuitive knowledge, and the quantum mind. These correspond with our fundamental need to contribute and to know something greater than us.

The seventh and final need, associated with Sahasrara chakra, located at the top of the head, is the need for expansion. The qualities of this chakra are enlightenment, spiritual connection and truth, consciousness, and bliss. From the moment a being is born, that being has a fundamental need to expand; to go beyond boundaries; and ultimately to experience him or herself beyond the physical and time-bound form.

In my experience, all human conflicts at their very core involve these fundamental needs: security, autonomy, authenticity, connection, beauty, meaning, and expansion. If in any conflict we are able to move from positions to exploration of these fundamental and universal needs, the very nature of the conflict changes. I imagine that at this point expansion from positions to interests, e-motions, values, and needs can feel quite abstract. We will explore some tools for generating this movement within ourselves and in conflict situations later, first let's see how this expansion may work in a controversial, charged, and highly polarizing issue.

The murder of George Floyd in Minnesota in the summer of 2020 reignited a highly charged debate in America on policing and the treatment by police of people of color. The two sides of this debate became defined by positional slogans—Defund the Police and Back the Blue. Let's take these slogans through the expansion spectrum—from positions to interests, e-motions, values, and needs.

The interests behind the Defund the Police movement include punishing the police for years of systemic abuse and discrimination directed towards people and communities of color. Another interest is a belief that instead of directing resources towards increased militarization of police, the resources would be better directed towards various social services that could actually help people and especially people and communities of color.

On the other side, the Back the Blue crowd sees police officers as being unfairly targeted for enforcing laws they did not create while having to make split-second, life and death decisions. The interests here also include the belief that police officers are between a rock and a hard place: either they don't enforce the law and thus don't perform the jobs they were hired to do; or if they perform their job in tense, fast-paced, and confusing situations, and something goes wrong, they will be thrown to the wolves—fired, sued, and even imprisoned.

Despite the differences in positions and interests, when it comes to e-motions on both sides of this issue, there are some similarities. Likely both Defund the Police and Back the Blue folks feel a combination of anger, sadness, frustration, and anxiety about the future.

Likewise, there will be similarities in values between the two groups. These values include: accountability, fairness, equality, and justice. Now there may be significant disagreement as to the exact meaning of these values to each group and there definitely would be very different strategies to accomplish these values.

I would venture to say that most fundamental needs of the two groups are the same. Both groups have the need for security—knowing that they will be safe dealing with each other and that there are clear rules of engagement. Likewise, there is a shared need for autonomy or self-determination, especially in tense situations. There are also shared needs for authenticity—showing up as they are in different situations without the other side making judgments and assumptions about them; connection and meaning—ultimately both sides are concerned about an important social issue that goes beyond themselves and want to be seen, respected, and appreciated. Of course, even if both groups agree on some of their fundamental values and all of their needs, they still have very different strategies for meeting those needs. However, strategy disagreements can themselves be expansive and create room for exploration and growth.

Actually, when the issue of policing and the treatment of people of color is examined through an expansive lens, it is hardly binary, and is in fact full of nuance. Really looking at this issue reveals multitude of complex questions, like: what are the goals of policing and who gets to determine those goals? How is the effectiveness of police measured, especially in the communities of color? How to deal with the intersection of policing and other social ills such as multi-level systemic racism, poverty, easy availability and prevalence of guns, gang violence, limited availability of health and mental health services, underfunded schools, and addiction? What would it take to make careers in law enforcement attractive for bright, community-oriented men and women, and especially men and women from underprivileged backgrounds and men and women of color? What values, skills, and tools should police officers be trained on? What are the actual needs and concerns of the particular community where the officers are serving? These questions do not have easy, one-size-fits-all answers. Sincerely examining these questions could bring both sides together creating room to expand from binary, "us" vs. "them" thinking, to open exploration of multi-dimensional, creative solutions that address needs, values, and interests of all involved.

The Practice of Expansion

There are at least two dimensions to the practice of expansion: inner and outer. We will begin with the inner. As we discussed before, tuning inward is itself a way to expand our awareness and to discover our own positions, interests, e-motions, values, and needs. Another way to expand is to remember how little we actually know in any situation. As Sadhguru often points out, regardless of how much we know, there is always going to be a limit to our knowledge, whereas our ignorance is boundless. In fact, the moment we utter the words "I know," we close and narrow ourselves. If we know, what is there left to learn? What if in our everyday life we started replacing the words "I know" (especially when it relates to other people and their experiences) to "I am open" or "I am here now"? Commitment to this simple practice is deeply transformative and is a powerful way to expand.

Another important way to expand from positions to needs is by practicing gratitude. I am not just talking about the corny-sounding "attitude of gratitude," but about cultivating deep gratitude for the very existence that makes our lives possible. If we could realize just for a moment that we as creation are inseparable from the creator, just as the drop of the ocean is inseparable from the ocean. This is hard to remember and focus on in moments of despair. In those moments, picking up a leaf, blade of grass, or a rock and closely looking at them, seeing the intricacy of their design and brilliance of their engineering and realizing that our own design is no less intricate, elegant, and brilliant. And remembering, even for a moment, that part of our design is resilience and enormous capacity for growth. Sikh mystic Yogi Bhajan captured the essence of gratitude I am talking about when he said:

> The purpose of life is to watch and experience living. To enjoy living every moment of it. And to live in environments, which are calm, quiet, slow, sophisticated, elegant. Just to be. Whether you are naked or you have a golden robe on you, that doesn't make any difference. The ideal purpose of your life is that you are grateful—great and full—that you are alive, and you enjoy it.

Of course, I realize that there are times of such deep despair when gratitude may not be accessible. In those times, the best thing to do to expand is to serve. Serving means we willingly put the well-being of another above our own. When we serve fully and unconditionally, not to get something, but to give ourselves fully, we naturally expand. Hospice physician and author Rachel Naomi Remen has a profound statement in her book *Kitchen Table Wisdom: Stories That Heal* about service which in my view captures the very essence of serving. Dr. Remen wrote:

> Helping, fixing and serving represent three different ways of seeing life. When you help, you see life as weak. When you fix, you see life as broken. When you serve, you see life as whole. Fixing and helping may be the work of the ego, and service the work of the soul.

I experienced the true power of service when I volunteered for Sadhguru's Inner Engineering program. Inner Engineering is Sadhguru's signature program which initiates the participants into a deeply transformative yogic practice called Shambhavi Mahamudra. Volunteers manage and execute every aspect of this program which demands preparation, precision, and significant commitment of energy and time.

When I received a call asking me to serve as the coordinator for the event which was less than two weeks away, I was hardly in a great place. My story was that my life was in turmoil: my consulting business was slow; Juliya and I were in the process of selling our home; our finances were tight; even my spiritual practice seemed to have hit a plateau; I was unclear about where to go next and was feeling as close to despair as I have felt in my life. Coordinating a complex event with sixty participants and nearly a hundred volunteers felt like the absolute last thing I wanted to do. Yet, when the call came something within me compelled me to say "yes, I will do it." As I was hanging up the phone, I told Juliya: "I can't believe what I just agreed to do." Preparations for the event completely consumed me— there was so much to do and so many seemingly little details to remember. During the four-day initiation I hardly slept more than four to five hours each night. The event venue was an hour away from where I lived and I had to be there an hour before the 8:00am start. The days were long and did not end until 10 or 11pm, as after the participants left we had to clean and prepare the room for the next day; clean the kitchen we used for preparing food; and meet to determine the next day's tasks.

At the conclusion of the program, after the participants left, we had a brief meeting with the volunteers to thank them for their service and to offer an opportunity to share something about their experience. As I looked around the room, my fellow volunteers seemed tired, and yet there was an unmistakable glow about them. Most volunteers had busy personal and professional lives outside of this event. They could have easily done other things with their time. As we went around sharing our experiences, one comment really stayed with me. It came from an accomplished engineer who spent the event volunteering in the kitchen. His volunteer assignment included cutting vegetables, food preparation, dishwashing, and kitchen cleaning. He said: "In just about everything I did in my life the one persistent question was 'what about me?' and the versions of this question: 'what can I get out of this?' 'how will this benefit me?'" he paused before concluding, "In volunteering the prevailing questions were 'how can

I serve' and 'what would be the most helpful thing I could do?' This shift from 'what about me' to 'how can I serve' felt powerful and liberating." This volunteer expressed so eloquently how I was feeling. Yes, physically, I was exhausted. Yet, I was not drained. On the contrary, I felt invigorated and inspired. Invigoration and inspiration are expansive feelings. When we shift our focus from ourselves—our likes and dislikes; our grievances and anxieties—to unconditional service, expansion happens.

The practice of the outer dimension of expansion is about asking questions. Asking questions, especially open-ended questions which arise from the space of genuine curiosity and begin with "what," "where," "how," and "why," is how we expand from positions to interests, e-motions, values, and needs. This is of critical importance as author and journalist Malcolm Gladwell has pointed out in his thought-provoking book, *Talking to Strangers: What We Should Know About People We Don't Know*. We actually know a lot less about other people than we think we do. To illustrate this point, let us do a little experiment. Take a look at a below list of incomplete words:

P _ _ N
TOU _ _
_ _ TER
S _ _ RE
AT _ _ _
CHE _ _
_ _ _ EAT

Take a look at these words and try to complete them to the best of your ability on a piece of paper. Do you think your word choices say something about you? What if I told you that the choices of someone I know were: PAIN, TOUGH, HATER, SCARE, ATTACK, CHEAT, and DEFEAT? Would you say that the person who made these word choices is depressed? In pain? Is scared?

I will share that actually I was the one who made the above word choices and I don't believe any of the above words are in any way descriptive of me or how I feel. When Princeton University social psychologist Emily Pronin asked people to complete a series of words with missing letters, nearly uniformly those completing the words said that their word choices were just *word choices* that did not reveal much about them. On the other hand, when Pronin invited people to comment on other people's word choices, those commenting were quick to come up with all kinds of evaluations and diagnoses. Pronin refers to this phenomenon as "illusion of asymmetric insight." In her insightful paper in the *Journal of Personality and Social Psychology* titled "You Don't Know Me, But I Know You: The Illusion of Asymmetric Insight,"[40] Pronin wrote:

> The conviction that we know others better than they know us—and that we may have insights about them they lack (but not vice versa)— leads us to talk when we would do well to listen and to be less patient than we ought to be when others express the conviction that they are the ones who are being misunderstood or judged unfairly.

I learned about Dr. Pronin's fascinating research from Malcom Gladwell in *Talking to Strangers*. Gladwell himself has a very thoughtful take on how little we actually know about other people. He wrote:

> We think we can easily see into the hearts of others based on the flimsiest of clues. We jump at the chance to judge strangers. We would never do that to ourselves, of course. We are nuanced and complex and enigmatic. But the stranger is easy.
>
> If I can convince you of one thing in this book, let it be this: strangers are not easy.[41]

So, if we start with the assumption that we actually don't know what is happening in other people's lives, and I would suggest we don't even fully know the people closest to us, asking open-ended questions to better understand a person and to move from positions to needs takes on critical importance.

Early in my career as a mediator two middle aged African-American women came to see me. They represented that they were cousins and roommates. The women no longer wanted to be roommates and sought mediation to help them work through the logistics of separating their living arrangements. Initially, it seemed like this was a purely transactional and a relatively simple case: determine what it would take to remove one of the roommates from the lease; figure out the timeframe; and resolve who takes which possessions with them. We were making progress, though both women seemed a lot more angry and sad about the situation that is typical of two roommates. That is until we got to the old couch of limited market value. Our progress halted at this point. Both women seemed attached to it, unwilling to move an inch, insisting that each should have it. "I paid for this couch with my own money! It is mine and mine alone! I don't care that you like it or you want it! Get your own damn couch!!!"—yelled one woman angrily. As her roommate heard this, a loud, primal sob escaped her chest. She began to cry as though she was a young child. Meanwhile, the other woman stared into the floor while biting hard on her lower lip. "Why don't we take a break?" I suggested, "so that I can check in with you individually." Both women nodded in agreement, while still lost in their emotions. To give some space to the crying woman, I first met with the other one. "Tell me more about this couch" I began gently. "Why is it so important?" After I posed my questions, long and thick silence ensued which I knew not to interrupt. "You know" the woman in front of me began slowly while meeting my eyes, "we are no roommates or cousins! She's been my lover, my partner, and my best friend for the past fifteen years! That couch was the first piece of furniture we purchased as a couple!" the woman finished with her voice dropping.

This was not such a simple case after all. Two "roommates" and "cousins" in front of me were not like that at all. They were life partners mourning the loss of a relationship. Their dispute was not about a couch. The old couch was just a symbol of a relationship lost. Asking open-ended questions and not assuming that I knew helped to uncover what's behind the couch and to move from positions ("I want the couch") to needs—needs for security, autonomy, authenticity, connection, and meaning. Besides the couch, the two women in front of me shared these needs. Identifying and meeting those needs was what our mediation was about.

10

EXPLORATION

My good friend, Adina Tovell, pioneered a brilliant term—courage to be curious. Courage to be curious is the best summary of the fourth principle of conflict transformation—exploration. By the way, if you are looking for a fun, inspiring, and insightful podcast, check out Adina's *Courage to be Curious* podcast.[42]

Exploration in conflict means we let go of our projections and limited ideas of what should be and allow ourselves to explore infinite possibilities that actually most conflict situations bring. Exploration is closely tied to expansion as exploration itself is an expansive process which can bring creativity, curiosity, and even excitement to conflict. Exploration in conflict is anything but natural or easy, as it requires us to lean into conflict instead of avoiding it. When we lean into conflict with courageous curiosity, we transform a destructive and draining interaction into an expansive and meaningful one.

In the book *High Conflict: Why We Get Trapped and How We Get Out*,[43] which I referenced earlier, Journalist Amanda Rippley uses a powerful example to illustrate how impactful leaning into conflict to explore different possibilities can be. Rippley talks about a prominent New York City synagogue called B'nai Jeshurun. Being over two-hundred years old, B'nai

Jeshurun, known to its members as "BJ," is one of the oldest synagogues in New York. BJ's imposing Moorish building is right off Broadway in the prestigious Upper West Side area of Manhattan. By virtue of its stature and location, BJ is home to one of the most influential Jewish communities in America. As Rippley describes, BJ came nearly undone when a controversy erupted in 2012 after the U.N. granted Palestine a non-member observer status. While largely symbolic, this change for the first time in history enabled Palestinians to participate in General Assembly debates. While many pro-Israeli and Jewish groups in America opposed the U.N.'s action, BJ's rabbi, an outspoken Argentinian named Jose Rolando Matalon, known as Roly, celebrated the UN's decision in a public email to his congregants. Rabbi Matalon's email generated quite a stir within his prominent congregation, resulting in a telling *New York Times* front-page headline, "Cheering U.N. Palestine Vote, Synagogue Tests its Members." Just a short time later another controversy erupted when Rabbi Matalon and another BJ rabbi, named Felicia Sol, publicly criticized the mayor of New York for his support of a powerful pro-Israel lobbying organization. In reaction to these controversies, a number of congregants who for years associated with BJ either left or were considering leaving, accusing BJ's leadership of being anti-Israel and even against Jewish people. As Rippley describes:

> These accusations cut Roly deeply. He had lived and studied in Israel. He'd organized countless educational programs on Israel and led many BJ trips there. The reason he criticized certain Israeli government policies was *because* he cared so much about Israel. And now he was being called "anti-Israel"? It was mind-boggling.

As the conflict among BJ's congregants escalated and people sorted themselves into "for" or "against" camps, Rabbi Matalon had three bleak options: to leave the congregation he loved and had dedicated nearly thirty years of his life to; to fight, so that those who disagreed with him left; or to censor himself, and stop sharing his personal views about Israel. As Amanda

Rippley describes, Matalon chose the fourth option, which proved to be transformative for him and his congregation. In Rippley's words:

> After months of agonizing, Roly agreed to a fourth option. He would not leave, fight, or surrender into silence. Instead, he would try to keep his congregation together by going deeper into conflict. "We leaned into it."

For BJ, leaning into conflict meant bringing in a specially trained mediator, Rabbi Melissa Weintraub, who was the cofounder of the dialogue organization called Resetting the Table. For months Rabbi Weintraub led BJ congregants into a deep exploration of the views relating to Israel they held. This exploration was profoundly transformative as through it the congregants discovered that their views on Israel were quite nuanced. More importantly, through many dialogue sessions facilitated by Rabbi Weintraub, BJ congregants were able to move from binary "us" vs. "them" positions to deep exploration of values and needs. As Amanda Rippley describes:

> It became clear that many people wanted the same end goal: for Israel to be stable and secure *and* for the Palestinians to have independence and dignity. What they disagreed about—profoundly— was how to get there.
>
> The other revelation was that there were not just two schools of thought. Some people took extreme positions but many more had ambivalent feelings. They struggled to reconcile it all. Their answers might be different from one day to the next, depending on how the question got asked. That's because there was no easy answer. The conflict was external as much as internal.
>
> Eventually, [the congregants] got to a place where they could express their own views *and* "tolerate the discomfort of someone else's opinion"...

For BJ congregants and Rabbi Matalon, exploration certainly was not easy. It required people to open up and soften, when it was much more natural to close and harden one's positions. Yet, the courage to be curious it took to lean in and explore this conflict not only expanded people's understanding, it transformed this community. As Rippley describes, following this conflict, BJ built a whole infrastructure for exploring differences, rather than avoiding conflict. This infrastructure included hiring Rabbi Weintraub, the mediator who led discussions relating to Israel, as one of BJ's associate rabbis. Another piece of this infrastructure included training congregants in active listening, which created space for greater understanding even when there were persistent and profound disagreements. BJ utilized this infrastructure time after time when conflicts erupted within the congregation. In fact, BJ used this infrastructure to address a controversy over interfaith marriage which erupted a few years after the Israel situation. In the marriage situation, the congregants once again leaned into conflict to explore what was behind divergent and seemingly binary positions to interests, emotions, values, and needs. Inevitably, this exploration brought more complexity and nuance to the situation. Ironically, more nuance and complexity also created space for better understanding, greater tolerance, and deeper connection.

In my own work, I've witnessed the transformative effects of exploration in many highly charged conflicts. When we are able to approach conflict with courageous curiosity and willingness to explore, there is generally a very palpable shift in the parties. If we are able to get to exploration, even if there are profound disagreements, there is a very high chance that the conflict will be resolved.

In my life, willingness to explore—to take an unexpected turn, to experience expansive risk—has had a powerfully transformative impact. As I discussed in Part I of this book, I would not be here, doing the fulfilling work I am doing or even writing these words, but for a motorcycle which took me on a different path in life.

Like tuning inward, observation without evaluation, and expansion, exploration is more of a guiding value or principle rather than a specific technique. Nonetheless, below we will explore some specific techniques of bringing courageous curiosity to conflict.

The Practice of Exploration

Like one of my mentors, Brad Heckman of the New York Peace Institute, when teaching mediation to students I often use a drawing of a DeLorean car to illustrate an important tool of exploration in conflict. DeLorean, a sports car made for only a few years in the 1980s, is synonymous with the cult classic film, *Back to the Future*. The skill of exploration I am illustrating with a DeLorean is future casting.

Future casting is about shifting the focus in conflict from past grievances to an exploration and vision for the future. When working as a mediator with divorcing/splitting couples, especially those with young children, I often invited them to write out their divorce/split up story from the perspective of twenty years from now, perhaps as they are sitting at their daughter's or their son's wedding. It was incredible to observe how this little bit of future focused exploration helped the couples to focus on things that were truly meaningful and important for them.

Another tool of exploration I use and illustrate with a picture of a unicorn and a rainbow is known in the field of facilitative mediation as ideal visioning. When I practiced law and especially in later years, after my exposure to Yoga and to various conflict resolution methodologies, it used to always irk me when judges expounded on the value of settlement, giving a clichéd explanation that a "good settlement is when everyone walks away being a little unhappy." What a terrible aspiration settlement presents! Instead of aiming for something where everyone leaves a little bit unhappy, I believe it is a lot more useful to start with everyone's ideal vision. When I pose a question to folks I work with in conflict: "In the ideal world, in the world of unicorns and rainbows, what would you like to happen in this situation?" most people begin with sharing vague generalities (i.e. "I just want peace" "I hope we can simply get along" "Is respect too much to ask???"). It often takes quite a bit of coaching to help people to be able to articulate a more specific vision. Once we are able to do that, I use that vision as a starting point in our conversation. We might not be able to get to someone's ideal vision and we don't always get all that we may want. Yet, why not start at the ideal place and then move from there?

The final tool of exploration I will share here is a way to utilize creative brainstorming. The key to creative brainstorming is to separate idea generation from idea evaluation. This enables us to get as many ideas up as possible without evaluating them. When working with creative brainstorming, I encourage folks to come up with as many ideas as possible, even if they are crazy, outrageous, or seemingly unworkable. I can't tell you how many times a seemingly crazy idea transformed a conflict interaction.

The best example of this comes from Brad Heckman, formerly of the New York Peace Institute. Brad was asked to do some organizational development work at a very large and complex governmental organization that shall remain nameless. It seems that at the time this organization experienced some climate issues where there was a generational gap—between seasoned workers who worked on some critical agency missions and the new generation of millennial professionals who saw the culture as too rigid and who craved a less formal work atmosphere, conducive of creativity and team building. In working with a group of organizational leaders Brad led a brainstorming exercise where he invited those present to share ideas without evaluating them, with a goal of getting as many ideas as possible on the whiteboard. One young manager brought up the idea of having a petting zoo. Now, if you think about the government and everything that it stands for, it is hard to imagine an idea more out of place. The young manager's colleagues laughed, seeing the idea as a joke and being ready to dismiss it. Brad gently reminded them that all ideas were welcomed and that now was not time to evaluate. Later, Brad took the opportunity to better unpack the young engineer's idea. Behind it was a strong desire to have some ways for releasing stress and dealing with the immensely high pressures and demands of the job. This idea led to further exploration—both of this agency's culture (did it need to be so high-pressure and stressed?) and other ways for dealing with stress and the job demands. While, as far as I know, this government agency did not end up having a petting zoo, the young manager's idea and the exploration which followed brought more nuance and better understanding of the underlying needs of the various groups in this very complex work environment. In other words, brainstorming without evaluating broadened the dialogue, creating more room for expansion, connection, and meaning.

11

THE SEED, THE ROOT,
AND THE FRUIT

At the beginning of this book, I used the analogy of the seed, the root, and the fruit. I'd like to revisit this analogy to place the preceding chapters and the parts of the book that follow in a proper context. Shifting our focus inward, rather than outside of us, is the seed. It is what ensures that we start showing up to conflict interactions with the increased capacity to respond, or to take the action appropriate for the situation from an undisturbed state. The capacity to act from an undisturbed state, irrespective of circumstance, dis-solves the most fundamental conflict there is—conflict between life and *us*. As Sadhguru often points out, at the source of this conflict are our perceptions of the three core problems: that we are not happening the way we think we should happen; that life is not happening that way we think it should happen; and that other people are not happening the way we think they should happen. Are there any other problems we have?

The first problem occurs as the result of our perception that our thoughts, emotions, beliefs, prejudices, and preferences are *us*. At the source of our problem with life is the idea that we are separate from life;

that life is something happening *to* us; something we need to figure out; attach a meaning and a label to; be coached at; and to succeed in. Our problem with other people arises from the fact that while we don't know ourselves, we think we know other people and thus the way they should be. Dis-solving conflict from within is about dispelling all of these illusions. By shifting our focus inward we gradually start to gain some control over our thoughts, emotions, and energies and thus start happening the way we think we should happen. We also start accessing insights about the very nature of life and begin to experience ourselves as life and not something separate and distinct from it. As our sense of Self expands, we naturally become more inclusive. Further, we realize how little we know about other people and the idea that someone "should" be a particular way drops, giving way to natural compassion or connection with another person's innate humanity combined with a deep knowledge that we could never truly be in their shoes. Gradually, we realize that we are not even separate from other people or for that matter from the world. Thus, we start seeing even their violence and violence happening in the world as an expression and reflection of what is happening within us. By the way, the above insights are not just new age-ish beliefs we pick up. We believe something we have not experienced. Thus, we may believe that we could scale Mount Everest. However, once we do it, we no longer believe that, rather we *know* that we can. Likewise, we don't believe in apples. Most of us have experienced apples and thus we *know* what they are, we don't need to believe in them! Dis-solving conflict with life is like coming into a dark room fearing a snake there and then turning on the light and realizing that what we thought was a snake is actually a rope. Once we experience such a realization we cannot go back. With these realizations which become deep knowing, the way we experience conflict and other dimensions of life radically transforms. As Rhonda Magee, Professor of Law at the University of San Francisco and internationally acclaimed thought leader on mindfulness and Social Justice keenly observed in her powerful book, *The Inner*

Work of Racial Justice: Healing Ourselves and Transforming Our Communities Through Mindfulness:

> Through personal mindfulness practices, we can begin to ground, heal, and ultimately transform our sense of self, no longer clinging too tightly to a narrow and isolated sense of "I," "me," "my wounds," and the collective pain-stories of "my people." We can begin to be able to infuse our experience of ourselves in culture, community, and context with a sense of the valid, often painful experiences of others. And as we take in more of the whole, we grow.[44]

For the seed to germinate, take root, and to eventually deliver the fruit, it needs the right combination of soil, sunshine, air, and water. The four principles of conflict transformation which we discussed in the previous section of this book: tuning inward, observation without evaluation, expansion, and exploration along with the practices attached to each of these principles provide the necessary environment for the seed to develop and grow. These principles and practices cultivate the values of awareness, humility, curiosity, and growth. It is these values that form the strong roots of our tree. These principles, practices, and values create a culture of transformational conflict. Transformational conflict expands our understanding, enriches our interactions and shines a light on areas of our lives that require attention, deep reflection and change. Transformational conflict transforms challenging interactions from being the sources of pain, division, and stress into opportunities for reflection, growth, creativity, and connection. As Mediator Kenneth Cloke points out:

> In facing our conflicts, opening our hearts, and locating the center of what is not working, we pass through to the other side, uncovering hidden choices and transformational opportunities that ask us to develop, grow, and learn more about our inner selves.

Of course, no tree exists in a vacuum. On the contrary, it is in the state of constant synergy with all that it comes in contact with. The tools discussed in Part IV of this book—compassionate communications, restorative practices, and mediation introduce constructive and transformative strategies for engaging with others, especially those we disagree with. With support from properly trained facilitators and mediators, these tools can empower one to develop conflict resilience, increasing the capacity for understanding, connection, and growth. Just as the tree which survives and thrives through multitude of conditions, compassionate communications, restorative practices, and mediation can enable us to respond to conflict interactions with strength, clarity, compassion, and ease.

The fruit at the end is sweet indeed! That fruit is justice which as defined by Rhonda Magee (with echoes from Dr. Martin Luther King, Jr.) as "love in action for the alleviation of suffering...[which] begins with our awareness of the present moment, extends through caring for ourselves, and shows up in the love we bring to our interactions with others and our responses to the social challenges of our time." Yes, it will take time and energy for the seed to grow into a resilient and strong tree which yields sweet fruit and generates a new generation of seeds. However, let us not forget the power of the seed. The root and the fruit are ultimately within!

Part Four

TRANSFORMATIVE TOOLS

12

THE LANGUAGE OF COMPASSION

In Chapter 7 we talked about all the different ways we express our violence. As language is how we express ourselves and communicate with each other, naturally our violence shows up through our language. Our everyday interactions are filled with binary, imprecise, static, absolutist, passive, and judgmental language which alienates others; contributes to our own state of depression, anxiety, and apathy; and destroys relationships that are meaningful to us. I couldn't agree more with the American psychologist Wendell Johnson who made this keen observation about our language:

> Our language is an imperfect instrument created by ancient and ignorant men. It is an animistic language that invites us to talk about stability and constants, about similarities and normal and kinds, about magical transformations, quick cures, simple problems, and final solutions. Yet the world we try to symbolize with this language is a world of process, change, differences, dimensions, functions, relationships, growths, interactions, developing, learning, coping, complexity. And the mismatch of our ever-changing world and our relatively static language forms is part of our problem.

If we are to communicate with each other in a non-violent way we need a different language—a language of compassion—a language of life!

One book that has had an immense influence on me and my work is Marshall Rosenberg's *Non-Violent Communications: A Language of Life*[45].

In his book Rosenberg pioneered a simple, but transformative idea—a communication framework based in compassion—a mutual giving from the heart. In fact, as the flow of compassion is so central to Non-Violent Communications, I often refer to it as Compassionate Communications. Non-Violent Communications, or NVC as it became known, has four components which Rosenberg describes as follows:

> To arrive at a mutual desire to give from the heart, we focus the light of consciousness on four areas—referred to as the four components of the NVC model.
>
> First, we observe what is actually happening in a situation: what are we observing others saying or doing that is either enriching or not enriching our life? The trick is to be able to articulate this observation without introducing any judgment or evaluation—to simply say to people what we either like or don't like. Next, we state how we feel when we observe this action: are we hurt, scared, joyful, amused, irritated? And thirdly, we say what needs of ours are connected to the feelings we have identified. An awareness of these three components is present when we use NVC to clearly and honestly express how we are.
>
> …[T]he fourth component is a very specific request…This fourth component addresses what we are wanting from the other person that would enrich our lives or make life more wonderful for us.

In sum, observations (separated from evaluations), feelings, needs, and requests are four components at the heart of NVC. A mother communicating with her child may use the four components of NVC by saying:

Sam, when I saw your soiled socks near the TV in the living room, I felt irritated. I have the need to have more order in the common areas we share. Would you be willing to put your soiled socks into the washing machine or keep them in your room?

I illustrate the NVC/Compassionate Communications flow through the following chart:

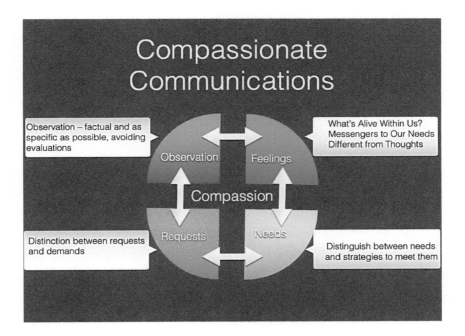

We've already talked about the transformative power of separating observations and evaluations. NVC does not require us to give up all evaluations, just teaches us to learn to separate the two and to refrain from moralistic judgements, binary labels, and unfounded conclusions. Especially when it comes to giving feedback to other people, NVC invites us to make our observations as specific as possible to time and place. To illustrate, let us do a quick exercise. It is similar to an exercise we explored before. This is an important skill worth reinforcing. Take a look at the phrases below and identify one which consists of an observation, as opposed to an evaluation, judgment, assumption, label or a conclusion:

1. "Deborah was angry with me for no reason."
2. "Omar has a big mouth!"
3. "During yesterday's meeting Kelly interrupted Rodney three times."
4. "La'Tonya did a great job in her presentation!"
5. "Jerri is often unprepared for meetings with me."
6. "When meeting with the patient last week, Dr. Brown listened to the patient without interrupting, and then reflected back what the patient had said."
7. "Morris is a real team player!"
8. "I think when we spoke yesterday, you were very unprofessional!"
9. "Aparna works too much!"

If you picked phrases 3 and 6 as those being observations, as opposed to evaluations, we are in agreement. Phrase 1 ascribes emotion to Deborah and assumes there were no reason for Deborah's emotion. Phrase 2 is a grotesque label which implies that Omar speaks too much. As this phrase tells us nothing about Omar's actual behavior, it is an example of a moralistic judgment. Phrase 3 is a clear observation. It is specific to yesterday's meeting and contains information that is as close to being factual as is possible (of course, without actually knowing what took place at yesterday's meeting between Kelly and Rodney). Phrase 4 is an evaluation (even though the phrase has a positive connotation). "Great job" is too subjective and imprecise to reveal any meaningful information about what actually happened during La'Tonya's presentation. Phrase 5 is also too imprecise and thus judgmental. Both the words "often" and "unprepared" are too vague to really reveal anything of meaning. Phrase 6, which as we established, contains an observation which is specific to time and tells us precisely what Dr. Brown did. Phrase 7, while positive, does not really reveal to us what Morris did to be seen as "the real team player." Because of the imprecision of information, it is an evaluation and a conclusion. In phrase 8, the word "unprofessional" is very vague and subjective. It is a label and not an observation. Likewise, phrase 9 contains a judgment as the meaning of "too much" is unclear.

I am going to hold off for a moment talking about feelings as this is where I respectfully diverge with Rosenberg, and will instead first cover needs and requests. Rosenberg utilizes a slightly different needs inventory than I do. However, fundamentally, everything I have previously said about needs is applicable here.

In many ways, requests are similar to observations in terms of their precision and specificity. Rosenberg uses a powerful question to illustrate requests—What would make life more wonderful for us? If that's the question, wouldn't we want to make the answer as specific as possible to make it easier for our conflict partner to make life wonderful for us? The below New Yorker cartoon brilliantly illustrates this very point:

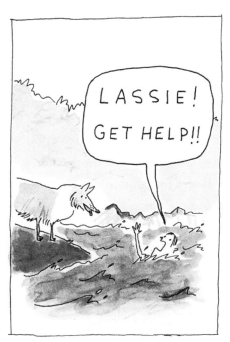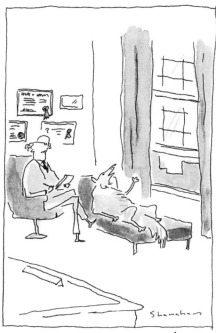

www.cartoonstock.com

"Lassie! Get help!!"—yells a drowning person to their dog on the shore. In the next frame, Lassie is getting "help" as she is shown laying on the couch at the therapist's office.

Vague generalities, lack of precision in language, passive voice, and not asking for what we need are ways in which we avoid conflict, often in the name of civility and collegiality. Rosenberg makes it clear that such avoidance strategies are yet another way we express our violence. Communicating in a compassionate and non-violent way means communications that are precise; specific to context, time, and place; and communications where we take absolute responsibility for our feelings, and ask for exactly what we need while being open to receiving feedback and requests from others.

Now let's get back to feelings. Like many trained psychologists, Rosenberg advocates developing a "feelings vocabulary" to be able to identify and to communicate what one is feeling. I would agree with Rosenberg that it is important to distinguish when we are talking about feelings as opposed to when we are evaluating or assuming. Thus, we are not talking about feelings when we use words such as "that," "like," and "as if". So, the following three sentences would not represent a feeling:

- "I feel that you should know better."
- "I feel like a failure."
- "I feel as if I'm living with a wall."

Likewise, when we use pronouns "I", "you," "he," "she," "they," and "it" to qualify our feelings we are also not referring to feelings. Accordingly, the statements below would also not represent a feeling:

- "I feel I am constantly on call."
- "I feel it is useless."

Finally, names or nouns referring to people also would not represent a feeling.

- "I feel Amy has been pretty responsible."
- "I feel my boss is being manipulative."

All of the above do not reflect one's inner experience, and thus are not talking about feelings.

Where I differ with Rosenberg is in specifically labeling the feelings we experience. This is a very common practice among psychologists, psychiatrists, and therapists. In fact, many mental health professionals utilize special charts or other tools to try to identify the feeling one is experiencing as clearly and precisely as possible.

As we discussed before, feelings are complex and multi-dimensional inner experiences, not easily reducible to a single word or phrase. For instance, someone may be feeling anger and confusion; or fear and anxiety; or even happiness and sadness (i.e. someone graduating from college may feel happy that they are finally done, excited about the next steps, and sad about no longer being able to spend as much time with their college roommate as they did before). Further, the words we use to describe feelings, such as anxiety, fear, anger, sadness, and apathy, have long had stories and conditioning attached to them. These stories and conditioning in turn stigmatize individuals who express these feelings, often along gender and race lines. For instance, there are stigmas towards women and Black and Brown people who express anger and towards men who feel anxious or sad. Most importantly, focus on the right vocabulary—the proper label—could actually mask the actual feeling.

This became abundantly clear to me during a very challenging mediation I was involved in. Jerry and Bob were two brothers in NYC who were struggling to take care of their ailing father, Harold. Jerry, the younger brother, was a trained psychologist and worked in the field of organizational development. Both Bob and Harold were prominent psychiatrists in New York, though Harold was long retired. Jerry and Bob specifically sought a mediator trained in Non-Violent Communications and a colleague referred them to me. When we met, Jerry was the first to speak. He shared that he was feeling sad about the fact that he and his brother could not agree on the best way to care for Harold, who, while exhibiting signs of dementia, was also fiercely independent. As I reflected back to Jerry what I thought I heard him say, Jerry informed me that he was feeling concerned that my reflection was not as precise as what he would have preferred. He requested that to satisfy his need for clarity I reflect his words more precisely. Welcoming Jerry's feedback, I agreed. Then it was Bob's turn to speak. Politely but firmly Bob pointed out that when Jerry spoke about his sadness, actually what he described was not sadness, but anxiety or fear. Bob shared that he was dismayed that his brother, despite being a trained psychologist, was not fully in touch with his emotions. He expressed a need for more authentic connection with Jerry and requested that Jerry identify his true feelings and needs. Jerry responded with just a slight irritation in his voice that he was very clear that he was feeling sadness, but now was also beginning to feel anger. He said that he also had a need to connect with his brother but believed that he was not being heard. He requested that Bob reflect back what he heard Jerry say.

This went on for a while. Polite to a fault, the brothers were arguing about what feelings they were expressing and gently correcting each other's and my sentence structures which failed to adhere to NVC flow which Marshall Rosenberg outlined in his book. I was feeling increasingly frustrated as nearly two hours into our session, we had barely spoken about Harold, Harold's condition, or his care needs. This was going nowhere! I decided to check in individually with each of the brothers, sensing that our session was not serving them just as it was not serving me. "Jerry, could we forget for a moment about NVC and the proper terms for feelings?" I started gently when I was alone in the room with him. "Could you just tell me what's going on?" I continued. Upon hearing my question, Jerry lowered his gaze and dense silence filled the space between us. While continuing to examine the intricacies of the industrial-grade carpet on the floor, Jerry spoke, softness and uncertainty in his voice: "I can't stand him!" he said while raising his eyes to meet mine. "Bob thinks he knows everything and he always has to be the smartest person in the room. What an asshole!" concluded Jerry with a lot more conviction, once again focusing his eyes on the floor. As we continued our conversation, I learned that Jerry perceived Bob to be the favored child by Harold, as Bob was disciplined and followed Harold in his footsteps into psychiatry, while Jerry took his time to find himself. As Harold was waning, Jerry desperately wanted his approval and wanted to be a part of his father's life while Harold still knew who Jerry was. He believed Bob was standing in the way of Jerry's relationship with Harold and was concerned that Bob was making all the decisions for Harold, increasingly isolating him from Jerry and other people who loved him and cared about him.

When I had time to check in individually with Bob, I began by posing a question to him: "How is it going, Bob? Do you think we are getting anywhere?" "I don't know," he began. "I think you're getting a Master Class on NVC. Rosenberg would be proud!" Bob said with a twinkle in his eye. After a pause he continued, "Look, Jerry wants to be there for the fun times, to see our father as his old, gregarious self. He doesn't want to be there when the going gets tough—when he soils himself or when he forgets his grandchildren," continued Bob as his voice dropped. As our conversation continued Bob revealed that he was always very close with Harold, following Harold into his career and eventually taking over Harold's practice. He was also geographically close, living just two blocks away. He believed that Harold's decline was much more dramatic than Jerry realized. He was frustrated that Jerry was simply not there to pick up the slack in taking care of their father's increasing needs. Bob also wanted a relationship with his brother, but saw Jerry as an unreliable and flighty partner who did not want to see or understand the full picture with Harold or how Bob was struggling to meet Harold's increasingly complex needs.

Eventually the conversation between Jerry and Bob became more productive. It took space for both brothers to tune inward and connect with their pain and to connect with the complexity, nuance, and ambiguity in the relationship between the two of them and each of their relationships with their ailing father. Through open-ended and very intentional questions; careful reflections where I could observe without evaluating, focusing on the emotion, energy, and intensity behind their words; and multiple caucuses where brothers could speak with me individually, out of the earshot of the other, we moved from entrenched positions, to interests, complex emotions, values, and most importantly, to needs. Finally, the brothers were able to openly explore various ideas for taking care of Harold and arrived at something both could live with. After four two-hour sessions, Jerry and Bob did not resolve all the issues between them. Yet, the energy in the room was far more easy going than during our first session. The brothers gently teased each other as they agreed to try out a caretaking arrangement for three months and then to check in with each other to see if any adjustments needed to be made. As we said our final goodbyes, I shook both of their hands. Bob held my gaze and said: "Thanks, Henry! Thanks for not letting us hide behind NVC!"

Jerry's and Bob's case revealed something profound to me. As a technique, NVC offers a powerful way for people to communicate with each other, yet it also has limitations. One can get too caught up in the technical application of the technique—in crafting sentences which follow the perfect NVC flow (i.e. sentence and paragraph structure which contains an observation, expression of a feeling and need and the making of a request). Such sentences, while mechanically correct, carry none of the intentions or impacts of truly non-violent and compassionate communications. In my experience, for NVC to work as intended, critical inner work must happen first. Truly connecting with our feelings and experiencing them fully, in all their ambiguity, nuance, and complexity is much more important than reducing them to a single descriptive word. Likewise, it takes time, introspection, and practice to be able to identify our needs and to make requests of others that truly serve our needs and demonstrate absolute willingness to consider the needs of others. As I connected with Rosenberg's work, saw its simplicity and inherent brilliance, it also became clear to me that there had to be a prequel to it. The previous chapters of this book provide this prequel. Communicating with others in a non-violent way is more than a sentence structure. It takes the experience, the practice, and the states of: tuning inward; observation without evaluation; expanding; and exploring.

13

RESTORATIVE APPROACH TO CONFLICT

For centuries, long before Western concepts of law and order and with it the system of binary adjudication—right vs. wrong—influenced societies around the world, Navajo and other indigenous people approached conflict based on very different principles. Western-based systems of conflict resolution utilize a "vertical" system, one which relies on power and hierarchies. Further, as Robert Yazzie, the former Chief Justice of the Navajo Nation pointed out:

> A fundamental aspect of the vertical justice system is the adjudicatory process. Adjudication makes one party the "bad guy" and the other "the good guy;" one of them is "wrong" and the other is "right." The vertical justice system is so concerned with winning and losing that when parties come to the end of a case, little or nothing is done to solve the underlying problems which caused the dispute in the first place.[46]

Justice Yazzie continued:

> Another element of the vertical system is a preoccupation with "the truth." The adversarial system dictates that there must be a winner

and a loser. The side that represents the truth as it is perceived by the court wins, while the other side loses. "Truth" becomes a game where people attempt to manipulate the process, or undermine it where it does not suit their advantage. Each person has a version of "the truth," which represents that individual's understanding or perception of what happened.[47]

On the other hand, the traditional Navajo system of conflict resolution is "horizontal," in that it sees all beings as being inherently equal. It sees conflict as something which requires healing, as opposed to a determination or resolution. As Justice Yazzie describes:

> A better description of the horizontal model, and one often used by Indians to portray their thought, is a circle. In a circle, there is no right or left, nor is there a beginning or an end; every point (or person) on the line of a circle looks to the same center as the focus. The circle is the symbol of Navajo justice because it is perfect, unbroken, and a simile of unity and oneness. It conveys the image of people gathering together for discussion.[48]

In fact, the Navajo justice system institutionalizes the custom of *hozhooji naat'aanii*, or peacemaking.[49] This custom utilizes a ceremonial process where disputants and community members gather to "talk things out" with the assistance of *naataanii*, a respected community member who serves as a peacemaker.[50] The *naataanii* assists all the individuals involved in the peacemaking process to reach consensus with the goal of returning individuals and the community to a state of *hozho*, or harmony.[51] The underlying vision of the Navajo approach is interconnectedness—the realization that "we are all connected to each other and to the larger world through a web of relationships. When this web is disrupted, we are all affected."[52]

The peacemaking tradition of the Navajo and other indigenous people provided the foundation for the Restorative Justice movement which has taken root in a variety of settings, such as criminal justice, education, and organizational development in North America, Europe, New Zealand, and beyond. Howard Zehr, one of the leading Restorative Justice proponents and scholars in North America, defines Restorative Justice as:

> ...a process to involve, to the extent possible, those who have a stake in a specific offense and to collectively identify and address harms, needs, and obligations, in order to heal and put things as right as possible.[53]

Zehr identifies four key features of Restorative Justice: inclusive decision-making, active accountability, repairing harm, and rebuilding trust.[54] While Restorative Justice involves a variety of different practices, one of the most common applications and the one I found to be very useful in addressing a wide range of conflicts is the Peace Circle. Peace Circles also most closely mirror the practices pioneered by the Navajo and other indigenous people.

Peace Circles

Peace Circle is one of the most powerful peacemaking practices with deep roots in the indigent tradition. In her book, *The Little Book of Circle Processes*, Kay Pranis, one of the leading teachers and facilitators of Peace Circles, expanded on the historical context of Peace Circles as follows:

> Peacemaking Circles draw directly from the tradition of the Talking Circle, common among indigenous people of North America. Gathering in a Circle to discuss important community issues was likely a part of the tribal roots of most people. Such processes still exist among indigenous people around the world, and we are deeply indebted to those who have kept these practices alive as a source of wisdom and inspiration for modern Western cultures.[55]

Peace Circles are a Restorative Justice practice now widely utilized in the criminal justice, educational, community building, and corporate arenas. Kay Pranis further describes Peace Circle as

> ...a story-telling process. Every person has a story, and every story has a lesson to offer. In the Circle, people touch one another's lives by sharing stories that have meaning to them. ...[S]tories unite people in their common humanity and help them appreciate the depth and beauty of the human experience.

This is rather ironic, as by being able to share our stories while listening to other people's stories in a safe and welcoming environment we are able to create space between our stories and us, thus transforming the conflict.

Peace Circle contains five critical elements: a Ceremony, Talking Piece, Facilitator/Keeper, Guidelines, and Decision-Making by Consensus. Circles "use a ceremony or intentional centering activity in the opening and in the closing to mark the Circle as a sacred space in which participants are present with themselves and one another in a way that is different from an ordinary meeting."[56] A Talking Piece marks who is speaking and ensures that Circle participants speak one-at-a-time, as only the person holding the Talking Piece speaks while everyone else listens. Facilitator/Circle Keeper is one among equals who "monitors the quality of the collective space and stimulates the reflections of the group through questions or topic suggestions." Mutually agreed-upon guidelines are critical to the success of the Circle as they articulate the shared commitment to "the behaviors that the participants feel will make the space safe for them to speak their truth." Finally, consensus, in the context of the Circle, does not mean that every participant must be enthusiastic about the decision or plan. However, it implies that each participant "is willing to live with the decision and support its implementation."

Recently, I had an opportunity to experience the power of the Peace Circle in action in a conflict involving highly charged identities.

A group of Jewish students at Virginia Tech had planned to hold an Israeli-themed Shabbat dinner. Thus, they hung an Israeli flag outside the student center where this event was to be held. A student of Palestinian origin was passing by and took offense to the display of the Israeli flag. He ripped the flag off and placed it in the garbage. This incident reverberated through the campus' Jewish, pro-Israel, and pro-Palestinian communities, re-igniting long-held narratives that both communities were quite attached to. My job was to facilitate a restorative Peace Circle among the impacted parties with the hope that the Circle would bring this incident to some kind of (hopefully peaceful) resolution.

I began by meeting individually with students who felt that they were impacted by this incident. In our individual meetings, I spent most of my time listening very deeply to the students. These deep listening sessions were of critical importance as they started the process of creating a safe space for the students' humanity to start to come out from behind the boundaries of their identities. In our listening sessions it became very apparent that these seemingly binary interactions were hardly so binary. Speaking about their experience, expectations, and feelings in a confidential, non-judgmental, and safe environment enabled the students to come to grips with the complexity of their feelings and the nuances of the overall experience. These listening sessions also helped the students to deal with the ambiguity of their expectations. What was really important to them? Was it retribution? Accountability? Some sense of justice? Security? Simply having a dialogue with someone they perceived to be their adversary?

After speaking with all the students who felt impacted by this incident, it was time to schedule a Peace Circle.

We began the Peace Circle with a Ceremony, where I lit up an oil lamp to honor anyone who has ever felt ostracized, excluded, or unsafe in our campus community and beyond. Since due to Covid we were doing this Circle virtually, we did not have a single Talking Piece. Rather, I invited all the Circle participants to bring in their version of the Hokie Bird. The Hokie Bird is a stylized turkey and the official mascot of Virginia Tech. It is also an important symbol of the Virginia Tech community, members of which refer to themselves as Hokies. As each of the students shared their representation of the Hokie Bird, I asked them to share what being a Hokie (i.e. a member of the Virginia Tech community) meant to them. When sharing their Hokie Bird and answering the question, the students talked about the importance of community; their sense of belonging; and support they received from other VT students as well as faculty and staff members. After everyone went around and introduced their Hokie Bird, there was a palpable difference in the virtual meeting room—there was a certain softness and a barely perceptible glow in the faces of the Circle participants. Restorative Justice Advocate, Peace Circle Trainer, and founder of New York's Restorative Center, Shailly Agnihotri[57] describes this palpable change as the moment when the Circle is formed. I then guided the students through co-developing the values for the Circle (equality, authenticity, and involvement) and the Circle guidelines (one person speaks at a time; no one ever has to speak, but if speaking be brief and speak from personal experience; what happens in the Circle, stays in the Circle). By the way, I did not invite the students to be respectful in the Circle. I did not want to impose my idea of respect on them. Also, in my experience, when everyone sees each other as human, respect is a natural consequence. It simply happens.

We were finally ready to talk about the incident and the multitude of complex narratives it revealed. The Palestinian student spoke first. He offered an apology to the Jewish students, explaining that he did not mean to target them. He also spoke of the myriad of complex emotions he experienced when he saw the Israeli flag—it was a reminder of the suffering his family endured in Palestine and the fact that while Jews had a country, he and his people did not. As the Palestinian student spoke, the Jewish students listened intently. When it was their time to speak, nearly every one of the Jewish students acknowledged the pain and ambiguity the Palestinian student felt. They also spoke of the shock of seeing the Israeli flag in the garbage can and the fear, apprehension, and anger they felt after this incident. We went around the Circle several times to ensure that everyone had a full opportunity to express how they felt and to respond to anything anyone else had said. Finally, I invited the students to brainstorm ideas for moving forward. The key here was that I asked them not to evaluate any of the ideas. The invitation was to generate as many ideas as possible, without evaluating them. After generating seven to ten different ideas for moving forward, we did a consensus building exercise to adopt one or two ideas into workable next steps. Students decided that they wanted to continue their conversation and to get to know each other better, first socially, so that then they could tackle more challenging issues between them. The students also agreed to exchange contact information so that they could coordinate events on campus and ensure that there were clear communications about symbols used. Finally, the students wanted to plan an event which honors all the different people which call Israel/Palestine their home.

In the grand scheme of things, and especially in the context of the complex and volatile Middle East Peace Process, the agreements the students reached were quite modest. However, I considered this Peace Circle to be a resounding success. The success of this Circle was not in any particular agreement or next step, rather it was in the transformation from binary, grotesque caricatures the students saw each other as before the Circle to the humanity, complexity, and nuance that the students experienced during the process. Behind this powerful transformation were four factors which we talked about before. These factors were: (1) tuning inward; (2) observation without evaluation; (3) expansion; and (4) exploration.

In meeting with me individually the students had the space to drop their guards down and thus to tune inward, becoming more introspective. The very structure of the Circle forced the students to observe more, while evaluating less. Narrow view of *us* and *them* expanded to a more expansive view of *us*—members of the same community, students, Virginia Tech Hokies. Finally, there was room for exploration—the students could approach their conflict with openness and creativity seeing multiple possibilities for building and repairing connections where there were none before.

14

MINDFULLY GETTING IN THE MIDDLE[58]

There is a *Seinfeld* episode where Elaine and Kramer are having a dispute over a bicycle. They both appeal to Jerry to resolve their dispute. Jerry waves them off, telling them that the fact that he is friends with both of them precludes him from getting involved. However, Jerry suggests that Elaine and Kramer use an impartial mediator, someone who has not heard the story before; and as Jerry states "someone whose heart is so dark, it cannot be swayed by pity, emotion, or human compassion of any kind." Jerry is talking about his archnemesis, Newman, who is all too happy to oblige in mediating the dispute between Elaine and Kramer. After hearing from both sides, and with all the pomp and circumstance befitting his important role, Newman delivers his decision: "we will cut the bicycle down the middle." As Elaine concurs, "yeh, cut the damn thing in half," Kramer interjects "let her have the bike!" he exclaims. This is where Newman delivers his true verdict: "only the bike's true owner would rather have someone else have the bike, than see the bike cut in half. Kramer, the bike is yours!"—concludes Newman. As the episode ends Kramer rides off on the pink bike, exclaiming "Sweet Justice!"

Of course, this Seinfeld episode satirizes the famous biblical story of King Solomon, which coined the phrase "split the baby in half." Unlike Newman in Seinfeld, King Solomon had to apply his wisdom to a more high-stakes dispute involving an actual baby. Though both sages, King Solomon and Newman that is, utilized identical logic, arriving at a similar result.

The Seinfeld episode and the biblical story on which it is based reflect the common perception of mediation—some wise character, unswayable by emotion of any kind, listens to both sides of an argument and then delivers some clever verdict, or at a minimum "splits the baby in half," forcing the parties to somehow settle, generally by meeting somewhere close to the middle. Many branches of the American judicial system and the field of the resolution of commercial disputes utilize a similar approach, known as evaluative mediation. Evaluative mediation involves a respected subject-matter expert, often a judge or an experienced lawyer, assisting in resolving a legal and/or commercial dispute. The goal of such resolution is often settlement and the expectation is that the expert mediating the dispute, who has no personal connection to the dispute, will evaluate the matter and suggest a reasonable result, at times pushing and at other times even coercing the parties towards the resolution the expert deems reasonable. As a lawyer, I've participated in a number of such mediation sessions, often known as settlement conferences. A similar version of mediation is utilized in foreign affairs. This is where respected, elder statesmen shuttle between parties in international conflicts, trying to win concessions, negotiate agreements, and achieve lasting cessation of active hostilities, if not full peace. Philosophically, these approaches to mediation view conflict as a fundamentally negative phenomenon, where the coolheaded mediator, "unswayed by emotion of any kind," can deliver an efficient cessation of hostilities through a negotiated settlement between the parties. As one judge shared with me and my client, sensing the client's reluctance to accept the resolution proposed by the judge, "a good settlement is where everyone is equally unhappy with the result." Settlement-based approach to mediation has relevance in the legal context, where it can free the time of overburdened courts and save the parties both the uncertainty and the immense cost of litigation. Further, in many commercial and even international disputes the relationships between the parties are purely transactional. In such situations, a settlement-based approach to mediation by a respected subject-matter expert could deliver clear, cost-effective, and legally sound results.

However, settlement-based approach to mediation in interpersonal conflicts and in disputes where the relationship among the parties is either ongoing or fraught with nuance and complexity raises significant concerns, brilliantly outlined by mediator Kenneth Cloke in his book, *Mediating Dangerously: The Frontiers of Conflict Resolution*, where he wrote:

> Mediators who seek settlement rather than resolution ignore the underlying reasons for the conflict, silence voices entreating to be heard, and plug up the transformational process. Mediators who seek to suppress conflict settle for half-measures, squelch honest ideas and feelings, and undermine the values that lie at the heart of the process.

Paraphrasing Robert Baruch Busch, one of the founders of the transformative mediation model, I see conflicts as crises in human interaction and thus see mediation as a process that helps the parties to regenerate and transform such interactions.[59] This shift happens when parties are able to move from compulsive actions, or *reactions*, to conscious ones, through which they are able to *respond* to conflict by strength, clarity and all-encompassing compassion. Thus, I fully adhere to Kenneth Cloke's vision of mediation. Cloke wrote:

> As mediators, we help people choose to surrender the illusions, mirages, and fantasies they have accepted about themselves, about others, and about their conflicts. We encourage them to recognize

a diversity of truths and to clarify and infuse their conflicts with meaning. We allow them to abandon stories that cast themselves as victims and others as demons. We assist them in recognizing their interconnectedness. We support them in overcoming their fears. We address their subconscious beliefs that if they admit their fears, they will be standing alone, naked, unprotected, and unsupported; that their compassion will lead them nowhere; that they will be unloved and unlovable. We aid them in moving to the center of their conflicts, where they can discover that reaching the center *anywhere* in their lives allows them to locate center everywhere.[60]

Thus, I define mediation as a conflict transformation process where a multi-partial mediator supports the parties in engaging in dialogue with each other without directing any particular outcome. This approach to mediation has four key goals which hopefully will sound familiar: to provide space for the parties to tune inward and to discover and/or clarify their positions, interests, emotions, values, stories, and needs; to offer an opportunity for clear observations without evaluations and thus ensure that the parties feel heard; to empower the parties to expand their understanding of the situation, themselves, and their own needs; and finally to explore complexity and nuance of the situation as well as possible outcomes. It is also worth defining the word "multi-partial," as many mediation practitioners and scholars prefer to use neutrality or impartiality. To me neutrality and impartiality sound sterile, dry, and legalistic, and create the impression that when serving as a mediator I leave my humanity at the door. In my experience, the opposite is true. I bring myself fully to the mediation process. Only by showing up as fully, unconditionally, and as centered as is possible for me can I create space for the parties to courageously move to their center and to tune inward, observe without evaluating, expand, and explore. So, I am a very partial mediator—I am partial to the process; and I am very partial to each of the parties as my intention is to create space, for everyone, myself included, to grow, connect, include, expand, and explore.

In fact, I see mediation as an integral part of living from within. I suppose it is fitting then that the origins of mediation are in the deeply spiritual practices from the indigenous traditions of Hawaii and Polynesia. The practice of *Ho'oponopono* is an ancient and integral part of Polynesian and native Hawaiian culture.[61] As indigenous people of Hawaii and Polynesia were expert sailors and fishermen, and also had a strong tradition of communicating through metaphors, the metaphor for conflict they utilized is entanglement, as in entanglement in the fishing net. *Ho'oponopono* thus is often translated as disentanglement or putting things as right as possible. Typically, *Ho'oponopono* had twelve distinct steps:

1. Gathering of the disputants by a "high status" family or community member who knows the parties
2. Opening prayer
3. A statement from the problem to be solved or prevented from growing worse.
4. Questioning of the participants by leader
5. Replies to the leader and a discussion channeled through the leader
6. Periods of silence
7. Honest confessions to the gods (or God) and to each of the disputants
8. Immediate restitution or arrangements to make restation as soon as practicable
9. Repeating the above steps as necessary to address all the problems and disputes among the participants
10. Mutual forgiveness by the parties of each other
11. Closing prayer, followed by
12. A shared meal or a snack[62]

While I do not strictly adhere to a singular mediation methodology, my approach to mediation has been primarily influenced by facilitative and transformative models of mediation. While there are distinct differences in the approach to mediation my colleagues and I utilize and the practice of Ho'oponopono, there are also some striking similarities. The model I generally utilize consists of the following ten steps:

1. Tuning Inward. This step consists of mediator's personal practice and also preparation for the mediation process, where the mediator intentionally attunes to the parties and their needs, to meet them where they are.

2. Opening.[63] In this step I introduce the parties to the mediation process, set expectations for possible outcomes and answer any process-related questions the parties might have.

3. Uninterrupted Time. During uninterrupted time each of the parties has an opportunity to share anything they wish to share about the dispute; their feelings; their concerns; or anything else they would like as I listen very closely to them, while attuning to the energy, emotion, and intensity behind the words.

4. Gathering Information. In this part of the mediation, the mediator engages with the parties by asking a series of questions to try to gain a better understanding of the parties needs and the issues involved in the dispute.

5. Setting an Agenda. Through setting the agenda the mediator identifies key broad themes among the parties to determine a path forward in their dispute.

6. Generating and assessing options. In this stage the mediator would assist the parties with generating and assessing options for moving forward.

7. Building an Agreement. In this stage the mediator assists the parties with building the final agreement.

8. Caucus. This stage of mediation could occur at any point and offers an opportunity for the mediator to meet individually with the parties.

9. Closing. In this stage the mediator would close the process, thanking the parties for their candor and participation.

10. Reflection. This is a critical stage of the process where the mediator would reflect on their approach and practice and make notice for future areas of improvement.

In utilizing these ten steps, I apply the following seven critical values:

1. Awareness. To the greatest extent possible, I maintain self-awareness. I do this by focusing on my breath and folding my tongue back (as I described when talking about active listening). Maintaining self-awareness throughout the mediation is what enables me to intuitively deliver what is most needed at the moment and to empower the parties to have the most meaningful interaction possible.

2. Authenticity. I have to show up to the mediation in the most authentic way possible for me. My absolute honesty, transparency, vulnerability, courage, and willingness to go deep is what creates the space for the parties to do the same.

3. Self-Determination of the Parties. It is always about the parties and meeting them where they are. The parties are in the driver's seat. I am merely the navigator, helping them to tune in, observe without evaluating, expand, and explore.

4. Safety. Physical and psychological safety of the parties is of paramount importance.

5. Movement Towards the Heat. The point of the mediation is not to avoid conflict, but rather to explore its full depth. Thus, respectfully and with the parties' permission, I always try to move towards the heat. Remembering the analogy from the beginning of this book, the fire alarm is the loudest as we move closer to the fire.

6. Confidentiality. For the parties to be able to have the most meaningful interaction possible, strict confidentiality is key. Even the courts recognize the importance of confidentiality in mediation

to allow the parties to communicate with maximum openness and candor and protect the confidentiality of all communications during a mediation through a doctrine known as mediation privilege.

7. Quality. I am committed to delivering the highest quality process for the parties. I am also committed to continuously improving my craft and growing on all levels and plains of my existence.

Jaden and Alyssa, a couple in their late twenties shared a small couch in the waiting area of my office. The close proximity of their bodies, their easy banter and interwoven hands suggested that they were really into each other. And, as if to dispel any doubt that they were lovers, right as I emerged from my office to welcome them the couple shared a passionate kiss on the lips. Giving them a moment, I gently cleared my throat before greeting them: "Alyssa! Jaden! It's great to see both of you! Why don't we all chat in the conference room?"

Alyssa had contacted me a week or so earlier at the suggestion of her father whom I casually knew through a professional organization we both belonged to. During our phone conversation Alyssa shared that she and Jaden have been seeing each other for about eight months and that things were getting serious. I also learned that Alyssa and Jaden both had relatively high-paying jobs—hers as a nurse anesthetist and his as a systems engineer. They were planning to move in together in the next month and had just put a deposit on a $500,000 townhouse in Philadelphia's Old City neighborhood. Alyssa had a five-year-old daughter from a prior relationship. The child lived with her. The child's father was not in the picture and did not pay support. Alyssa's father suggested mediation to Alyssa as he was concerned that Alyssa and Jaden were on different pages when it came to financial decisions. Alyssa thought her father's concerns were overblown, but shared with me that Jaden contributed one-third of the down payment for their new house, whereas she has contributed two-thirds. Jaden told Alyssa that one-third was all he could do right now. As Alyssa had the money, she did not press Jaden. Alyssa was assuming that once they moved in together, they would function as a family and share all expenses for the three of them from a "common pot." I asked Alyssa if she shared her assumption with Jaden and she told me that she had not. I also asked her if Jaden would be open to participating in a mediation with her. Alyssa told me that she had not discussed this with Jaden, but thought that he would be open to the idea, though probably would not be crazy about it. I shared some general information about mediation with Alyssa and invited her to speak with Jaden about participating in an introductory session with me. A few days later, Alyssa sent me a quick email saying that Jaden agreed. I scheduled the first available two-hour slot to meet with them. That is how Jaden and Alyssa found themselves cuddling in my waiting room.

Approximately fifteen minutes before my session with Alyssa and Jaden, I meditated and did some intentional breathing exercises, similar to the ones described earlier in this book. This is my regular practice before every meditation session. It enables me to be as present as possible with the parties and to tune in as fully as possible to where the parties are. As part of my usual practice, I also prepared the small conference room where I would be meeting with Alyssa and Jaden. Ideally, I like to have space for mediation that is not too large, is enclosed for privacy, and has some natural light. I also like to have another separate room where I can meet individually with the parties and where the parties can have a quiet and safe space to reflect, away from curious ears and the prying eyes of passers-by and as far as possible from all the sounds and commotions of a typical office. During the time of Alyssa and Jaden's mediation, I was sharing an office with a law firm. Thus, my space arrangements were not ideal. I had access to a smallish conference room which did not have windows. The door and one of the walls were made of glass, and accordingly were completely see through. In preparing the room for Alyssa and Jaden I set their seats in a way that ensured that they had their backs to the door. With the space constraints I had, this was a small measure of privacy that I could provide for them. I placed some fresh fruit in a bowl in the middle of the oval conference table along with a pitcher of water and two glasses. I also put a small bouquet of flowers on the side of the room's credenza. I brought fruit and flowers to enliven the space and to subtly remind myself and the parties of natural creativity, elegance, growth, and beauty so abundant in nature. The water was there for the convenience of the parties and also as a reminder of the flow of life. I was dressed casually in jeans and a sweater in the hope of communicating comfort to the parties and to de-emphasize my importance.

As Jaden and Alyssa settled into their chairs, while still clutching each other's hands, I sensed their anxiety. "Thank you so much for making the time to meet with me," I started as I smiled and made eye contact first with Alyssa, who smiled back and then with Jaden, who lowered his eyes to avert my gaze. "Do either of you know anything about mediation?" I continued. "Not really!" said Jaden as Alyssa vigorously shook her head. "Would it be helpful if I talk a little bit about the process—what you can expect and my role?" I continued in a soft voice. Both bowed their heads in agreement. I proceeded to briefly explain the mediation process, emphasizing confidentiality, the voluntary nature of the process, and the limited and multi-partial role I would be playing in whatever conversation Alyssa and Jaden were about to have. After concluding my brief soliloquy, I checked with both Jaden and Alyssa to see if they had any questions, which they did not. I then turned to Alyssa—"Alyssa, so, you contacted my office to request this mediation. What brings you here?" After posing this question I remained silent, to give Alyssa space to compose herself. A tense and long pause ensued as Alyssa dislodged her hand from Jaden's, laid her hands on the table and examined her manicured nails. "Jaden and I really love each other and we are excited to move in together," began Alyssa in a soft voice addressing no one in particular. She paused and then lifted her gaze to meet mine, and finding reassurance she was seeking, Alyssa's voice gained strength: "As we are putting our lives together, I wanna make sure that..." her voice trailed off as she paused "that we are on the same page financially and that Jaden accepts my daughter, who's the most important person in my world, and that he knows that we come together as a package!" rattled off Alyssa almost in a single breath as if she wanted to get all of this out before changing her mind. As Alyssa was speaking I took no notes, but instead made sure to watch both her and Jaden. Jaden's face revealed little in the way of emotion and his gaze was mostly glued to his folded hands. I noticed just a slight rise in his shoulders and a slight side-to-side head movement at the mention of Alyssa's daughter. When Alyssa was done I reflected back what she said, being sure to capture both her emotion and her intensity: "Alyssa, you and Jaden really love each other and you are excited to move in together! But…" I paused. "You would like to make sure that the two of you are on the same page financially." I paused again. "Most important for you," I continued "is knowing that Jaden accepts your daughter. Your daughter is the most important person in your life and you come together as a package! Did I hear you right, Alyssa?" "Yes!" she said softly though with conviction in her voice. "Jaden, you've been so patient! What brings you here?" I said as I turned my gaze and attention to Jaden. "I don't know why we are here!" he said, his voice rising with animation. "I mean, Alyssa wanted to talk about money. I think everything is pretty clear! We both make enough money to take care of ourselves and that's just the way it needs to be—we each take care of ourselves, and as far as I'm concerned, each of us could do whatever we want with our own money!" Jaden paused to catch his breath and then continued: "And, I'm sorry but her child, financially speaking, is her problem!" he finished. As Jaden brought up Alyssa's child, her mouth went agape and she rolled her chair to be further away from him. "My child is not my *problem*!!!" interrupted Alyssa "she is a part of *me!*" exclaimed now visibly upset Alyssa. "Alyssa, I know you feel very strongly about your daughter being part of you." I interjected. "Would it be ok if I reflected back what Jaden had said and then got back to you?" "Whatever!" Alyssa waved her hand dismissively, her eyes welling up with tears. "Jaden, you are not sure why you're here! It was Alyssa's idea to talk about money. As far as you're concerned, everything is clear: you each make enough money and you're both responsible for your own needs, and Alyssa is financially responsible for her child. Did I get this right?" I continued while keeping an eye on Alyssa. "That's right!" responded Jaden. Sensing that Alyssa was not really listening to Jaden and was getting too upset to continue, I decided to break in order to speak with the parties individually. This is the step of the mediation known as the caucus. I talked about the caucus at the beginning of the mediation and reintroduced it to the parties: "Hey, folks! You recall at the beginning of our time together I mentioned that from time-to-time I may ask to speak with you individually. I think now might be a good time for us to do that. So, we started this mediation with you Alyssa, how about I speak with Jaden first now?" I said, hoping to give Alyssa some space to reflect on what she heard and to compose herself. "Jaden, why don't you come with me to my office, while we let Alyssa hang here." as I motioned for Jaden to follow me. Once we were alone and sitting next to each other I asked Jaden how things were going for him. "Not so great," he responded with his big brown eyes locked in with mine. "She is upset now. I don't know if this was a good idea!" I dutifully reflected what Jaden had said, ensuring that he felt heard. "Jaden, I could be wrong, but I think I noticed your shoulders go up and you gently shaking your head from side to side when Alyssa brought up her daughter. Would you feel comfortable sharing with me what was going through your mind?" Jaden took a moment before responding: "Having a child freaks me out. Man, I don't know if I ever want to be a father. I am not sure that now..."there was a long pause, "I'm ready to be a father to a young girl who is not mine!" Jaden concluded as he once again lowered his gaze. "But, I really love Alyssa." Jaden continued unprompted. "I'm not sure what to do!" he implored. "Have you ever shared with Alyssa how you feel about having a child?" I asked Jaden. "No," he said. "Jaden, I invite you to think about how you could bring up how you feel to Alyssa. Perhaps this is something we can work through during the mediation. Also, Jaden, I invite you to think about what is important for you in your relationship with Alyssa." I paused and then continued: "Do you feel comfortable continuing with our session?" "We are here, we might as well," Jaden responded. Not exactly a ringing endorsement, but enough for us to continue. I left Jaden alone for a bit and returned to the conference room to speak with Alyssa. Her eyes were red from crying, but otherwise she seemed composed and was messaging someone on her phone. "How are you doing, Alyssa?" I started. "I'm OK," she responded. "I just need him to understand that my daughter is not going away somewhere! I'm not expecting him to pay child support or anything, but I want the three of us to be like a real family!" she continued unprompted. "Alyssa, in the ideal world, what does a real family with Jaden look like to you?" I asked. After contemplating for a bit Alyssa continued: "I don't know," she paused. "Doing things together, not feeling like if we go out together to get pizza I need to reimburse Jaden for Luna's slice." I noticed that this was the first time Alyssa referred to her daughter by name, so I followed up by asking "Could you tell me more about Luna?" Alyssa lit up. She was now a proud mother talking about her daughter. "Luna is a fun kid! She is five going on twenty. She is talkative, sassy, and artistic. I don't know where she gets all of this from!" concluded the now smiling Alyssa. "Has Jaden spent much time with you and Luna?" I asked. "Not really, he saw her once when picking me up at my mom's house." Alyssa responded. "In terms of building a family with Jaden and Luna, Alyssa, I'd like to invite you to think about what exactly would you want Jaden to do and the best way you can communicate that to him," I continued. "Sure," responded Alyssa. "Alright, how about I bring back Jaden and we'll do some more work together?" "Alright," Alyssa acceded.

When Jaden got back to the conference room, I asked Alyssa and Jaden to talk about their respective families (Alyssa was the youngest of four siblings in a close knit family where everyone was in each other's business and everyone shared everything. Jaden was the only child, raised by an immigrant single mother) and about how they met (through a singles website). As we were an hour and forty minutes into our session, I was sensing that Jaden and Alyssa were getting tired. I checked in with them if they wanted to pause and both agreed that they did. As I was thanking both of them for coming and made it clear that it was up to them if they wanted to continue with our sessions, Alyssa interrupted me and addressed Jaden: "Jaden, I hope we can continue talking. This was hard, but I hope we can continue talking. Today, though, I'll take an Uber to my mom's house. I've got some thinking to do," she said. Although Jaden tried not to show it, he was crushed. It was clear that both Alyssa and Jaden needed some space so I concluded the session by thanking them both for coming. I then sat in the room by myself and spent the next half an hour meditating and reflecting on what transpired. It was Jaden who contacted me a few days later requesting another session.

I could write another book just describing all the ups and downs Alyssa and Jaden had over the four mediation sessions which followed over the next three months. Through our sessions, both of them were able to tune more into what was truly important to them. By modeling active listening to them, I noticed that by the third session they were emulating me and listening better to each other. Their positions expanded, revealing nuance, complexity, and the ambiguity of their interests and emotions, and the similarities in their values. Of course, their fundamental needs—for security, autonomy, authenticity, connection, meaning, and expansion—were exactly the same, though Jaden and Alyssa were conditioned to meet their respective needs in very different ways. And Jaden and Alyssa explored various ways they could meet their needs. First, they proceeded with the purchase of the house. Also, they agreed that Jaden would spend more time hanging out with both Alyssa and Luna so that Jaden would see what it was like having a child. They also decided to pay all of their household expenses from a joint account and to maintain separate accounts from which each could spend up to five thousand dollars without seeking approval from the other. These agreements were not firm. Rather, Alyssa and Jaden agreed to try things out and keep checking in with each other to see how things would continue to evolve. These agreements were also not that important. Much more important than the agreements was the willingness of this young couple to have a difficult conversation with each other, leaning into conflict instead of trying to avoid it. During our last session I noticed a palpable difference in Jaden and Alyssa. While their public displays of affection were a lot more subdued, they were sharing a new level of intimacy with each other. I asked them what would happen down the line if they once again had a profound disagreement with each other. Jaden, who became a lot more expressive as we went through the sessions and grew much more comfortable with the process, said with a warm smile: "Then, we'll have to come back to mediation!" As we were concluding the session, I invited Alyssa and Jaden to share any last feelings, comments, or concerns that were arising for them. "This was difficult," Alyssa started. "But, I feel like I know better what is important for me. If Jaden and I could get through this, then Jaden, Luna, and I can get through everything!" she finished. Jaden took a moment before speaking. "Henry, I hated our first session and I hated you, because I thought this mediation would break up our relationship." He paused to contain rising emotion continuing as he regained his composure: "But then I thought if not now, then when? If not with the mediator, then how are we ever going to have these conversations?! This was powerful and important. I realized today that we came in here as lovers, and are leaving today as partners."

I share Jaden's and Alyssa's story to show that mediation can be messy, challenging, and nonlinear. This is a difficult process which can push the mediator's and the party's every button. Not every case ends the way Alyssa's and Jaden's did. Yet, this process also can be powerfully transformative for the parties and for the mediator.

To the critics of this approach to mediation who might be concerned that it veers too closely to therapy, I say that I perceive fundamental differences between the two. Often, therapy begins with a goal—to preserve the relationship; to improve communications; or to get through a difficult patch. Moreover, therapists often assist individuals or couples in analyzing, understanding, and shifting behavioral patterns. In mediation, conversation itself is the end goal. By enabling the parties to have whatever conversation they wish to have without the pressure of achieving any particular result, the mediator is empowering the parties to develop their own goals and measure their progress in moving towards or away from them. Likewise, mediators are not all that concerned with analyzing behavior patterns. Of course, we notice them and deal with these patterns only to the extent that these patterns impact the communication between the parties in conflict. Nor are mediation and therapy mutually exclusive. On the contrary, individuals, couples, and even groups of people could be a lot more effective in mediation if they are also working individually and/or collectively with an experienced therapist. Finally, the very unfortunate issue with therapy is the stigma attached to it. There is an assumption that something must be wrong for people to seek therapy. Perhaps because mediation is still much less known, there is less of a stigma attached to it. My personal sense is that Alyssa and Jaden would have had a much harder time sitting in the office of a professional counselor, psychologist, and/or marriage and family therapist than they did sitting in the office of a mediator. I have no idea if the end result would have been the same.

Ultimately, this book is about empowering people to have difficult conversations with each other, whether such conversations deal with global issues or with very local interpersonal disputes. The inner work outlined in parts one and two of this book enables people to come to the table more aware, more tolerant, more inclined to listen, and less likely to react to triggers with fear, avoidance, or aggression. Tools like compassionate communications, restorative practices, and mediation empower people to respond to conflict with strength, with clarity, and with ease once they are at the table. Therefore, these practices are integral for living from within.

15

SO WHAT, THEN WHAT

We are coming to the point in the book where an astute reader may be saying, "so, what," and "then, what?" "So, what, Henry, you have an interesting story. The tools and skills you offer may be useful for some self-improvement. They may even help with some interpersonal interactions, but then what? Does any of this have anything to do with the profound divisions and deep polarization we currently face? I still don't know how to talk to my cousin who is knee deep into conspiracy theories and seems to be living in an alternative reality; I don't know how to interact with people on social media where name calling and insults are the norm; and I am dreading Thanksgiving as I am just hoping to avoid blue/red, vax/anti-vax, he won/he lost shouting matches. Yet, there is only so much we can say about mashed potatoes! And, how does any of this help to address larger issues we face in the world. Will we meditate ourselves out of looming environmental disasters; systemic racism; growing divides between 'haves' and 'have-nots'? For crying out loud, we can't even agree on whether to wear a mask in the midst of a global pandemic!?"

These are legitimate questions that go to the very heart of this book. Is this another East meets West, New Age, self-help treatise which supposes to have all the answers, but offers little more than a few instagrammable quotes? The above questions reveal immense pain and also point to the profound collective fatigue with seemingly ever-increasing challenges, violence, and cruelty facing the world and with constant fearful and angry "us" vs. "them" fights.

These challenging times, however, also offer an immense opportunity—to fundamentally change the way we perceive ourselves and the world. Early on in this book we talked about mice paradise. It is worth revisiting the critters as we are moving closer to the end. Researchers at Emory University exposed a group of male mice to a mild electroshock while associating this painful experience with the smell of cherry blossoms[64]. While this experience was unpleasant, it did not result in any genetic changes in the mice. The male mice then mated with females producing offspring. Although the offspring were never exposed to either electroshock or the smell of cherry blossoms, they demonstrated stress behavior when exposed to the cherry blossom smell. This was still true even for the next generation of mice, where neither parent had any direct exposure to the electroshock and the associated smell. To control for possible ways mice could socially pass on the information, scientists eliminated any direct contact between the males exposed to the shock and smell and the females, inseminating the females in-vitro.[65] The result was the same—at least two generations of off-spring demonstrated stress response when exposed to the cherry blossom smell. This experiment demonstrates that we and mice (remember, we share over 90% of our DNA) are connected with each other across generations in ways which go beyond social interactions and even beyond genetics. In other words, what impacts one, impacts all. As physicist Werner Heisenberg wrote:

There is a fundamental error in separating the parts from the whole, the mistake of atomizing what should not be atomized. Unity and complementarity constitute reality.[66]

Physician, sociologist, and TED speaker Nicholas Christokis concurred when he said:

> We are, first of all, not solitary creatures and second of all, we are deeply embedded in the lives of others. It's very easy to forget that and to engage in an atomistic fallacy—where we think that all we have to do is study the individual components of a system in order to understand the system. That's clearly not the case when it comes to social systems.[67]

If we accept even for a moment the possibility that each of us is not an island, separate, disconnected, and distinct from everything and everyone, but an integral, connected part of the whole, then how we are and how we show up to life matters beyond mere self-help and personal growth. My hope is that one key takeaway from this book is that by tuning inward we can fundamentally change how we are and how we show up to the world. By changing how we are, we develop the capacity to respond to triggers, challenges, and conflicts with strength, clarity, and ease, instead of reacting to them with fear, avoidance, or aggression.

Anand Mehrotra taught a profound life lesson when in one of his discourses he said that attention is the currency of life. He added that wherever we place our attention, that will grow. Placing our attention outside of us increases the influences of outside factors—people and circumstances outside of us start having an outsized influence on us. This is especially true of those whom journalist Amanda Rippley refers to as "fire starters" and "conflict entrepreneurs". Fire starters and conflict entrepreneurs are individuals, organizations, and whole enterprises which intentionally or unintentionally sow division among us. They sow such division by triggering us and thus making us incapable of responding, and by reducing complex issues and multidimensional people into simple black and white, victim/victor, "us" vs. "them" narratives and caricatures. Consistent exposure to such narratives and caricatures contributes to biases and hatred and our experiences of anxiety, fear, and anger, as well as the sense of hopelessness and helplessness which permeates our lives. It is only by shifting our focus within, not as an occasional exercise in stress management, but as a way of life, that we begin cultivating and growing what is inside of us. What is inside of us is an infinite field of silence, access to wisdom, and ability to respond as opposed to react. More importantly, by shifting our focus within we start developing a distinction between what is *ours* and what is *us*. When I was in India I did a powerful meditation. The crux of the meditation is to keep inquiring "who am I?" At first, this meditation seems deceptively simple as we start it at the most superficial level—I am not these clothes that I am wearing, because yesterday I wore something different and *I* was still here. Now, how about my possessions beyond my clothes? Well, I am not my car, my motorcycle, my house, or my computer. As much as these items may enhance my life, I would still be here without any of them. How about less tangible items I've gathered? Well, actually I am not even the information, beliefs, prejudices, likes, or dislikes I've gathered. After all, there was a time in my life when I did not have this information; when I had different beliefs, prejudices, and preferences, and yet *I* was still here. Now, how about all of my personal and professional roles—college administrator, lawyer, teacher, son, husband, parent? Actually, throughout my life, my personal and professional roles have changed. Before I became a husband, a parent, or a lawyer, *I* was still here. Well, am I my thoughts? After all, French philosopher René Descartes famously said: "I think, therefore I am." However rare, I've experienced times in meditation when I did not have thoughts, and yet, once again *I* was still here. So, while I think a lot, I am not my thoughts. This is where we get to the really challenging part as we ask the question, am I this body? Well certainty, I've experienced life only through this body. It seems that before this body, I was not here, and will not be here once the body drops. But, hold on a minute, it seems that I am more than just a sack of skin holding some blood, bones, and body parts. After all, if you knew everything there was to know about my body, if you saw a detailed three-dimensional image of every organ, knew the chemical composition of my blood, saw detailed dissections of my heart, lungs, and even brain, you still wouldn't know *me*. And, when I die, you will make a distinction between Henry and his body, because while the body will be there, what animated this body, what made this body into a person you knew as Henry would be gone. So, then I am not just this body! There is something more to who or what I am!

This realization is one of the critical reasons why we look within and it has profound implications on how we relate with other people, especially those which trigger us or those we disagree with. So, let's get back to the question of how tuning inward can help us relate to the cousin steeped in conspiracy theories. In other words, how does focusing within help us have a more pleasant Thanksgiving?

First, if we realize that we are not the thoughts, beliefs, prejudices, preferences, and information we carry, then we also cannot reduce cousin Jeremy or other dinner guests to their political beliefs, views on the Covid vaccine, or to their opinions about past elections. There is so much more to each of us than any of this! Moreover, the more inward focused we are, the less we will identify with any particular identity, political or otherwise, as we will realize how little we know in any given situation. My teacher shared a beautiful story with me that illustrates just this. In ancient India, an elephant was often a much revered and honored domestic pet. One such elephant lived in an ashram. Six blind youths from a small Himalayan village came to the ashram to study with the ashram's Master. The youths have never encountered an elephant before. Upon their arrival at the ashram, the Master directed them to clean the elephant and then left to conduct business in town. Considering how large the animal was, one youth was cleaning the trunk; another youth the tail; and then four were washing the legs. After some time, the Master came back and asked the youths "So, what is an elephant?" The youth who cleaned the trunk shouted "It is this thick, elastic thing that's kind of like a rope." The youth who was cleaning the tail interjected, "Like a rope! No way!!! It sure is elastic, but is thin and small, kind of like a string." This is where the four youths who cleaned the legs began shouting in anger, "You two must have smoked hashish instead of cleaning and dreamed up your ideas! Elephant is not like a rope, or a string, it is like a thick tree trunk that can barely move." So, now there was a majority view and at least one conspiracy theory. Meanwhile, the youths were escalating their fight, shouting insults and waving their fists as the Master observed in silence. Finally, the Master stopped the youths with a curt "Enough!" followed by a period of silence as the youths were uncertain what to do next. After a while the Master spoke. "Each of you is absolutely right," he said and then paused again. "And each of you is absolutely wrong!" he finished. Through this tale, I am not suggesting that we don't know anything and that everything is relative, but we know for certain a lot less than we think. And we certainly know a lot less about people than our diagnosis, labels, evaluations, judgments, and conclusions make us believe.

Second, shifting our focus inward will increase our capacity to understand another being even if we abhor their views. By tuning inward ourselves, we can create a safe space for them to tune inward as well, to realize what is really important for them. We can observe without evaluating and engage in active listening. Utilizing the tools and skills we discussed we can expand from positions, to interests, to emotions, values, and finally needs. By expanding to needs from positions, we can see that even the needs of those we see as our archenemies are not different from ours. Finally, we can lean into conflict by exploring the possibilities our disagreements may bring. Even if we agree to disagree, this changes what our disagreements might look like, inviting us to focus on the important questions: how do we remember our humanity in conflict? How respectful conversations look and feel; and how do we ensure that everyone feels heard? All of these are powerful questions to explore to move away from the binary understanding of conflict to a place where we can engage with details and nuance. Where appropriate, you could utilize Compassionate or Non-Violent Communications, Restorative

Practices, or Mediation to create space for further understanding, expansion, exploration, and inclusion.

Third, there will be situations where it will not be possible or productive to engage with others. In fact, the *Yoga Sutras* by Patanjali teach us to be indifferent to the wicked. The wicked are not bad people, they are those who are so lost in their story and so rigidly bound within the confines of their identity, that interactions with them become both pointless and toxic. With people and entities like this, focusing within enables us to see them as they are, let go of the need to change them, and to let them be, while still seeing the humanity in them and feeling absolute compassion for their experience. With those who actively spew hate and contribute to division, I try to remember the words of writer, activist and civil rights leader, James Baldwin who wrote: "I imagine one of the reasons people cling to their hates so stubbornly is because they sense, once hate is gone, they will be forced to deal with pain."[68] Remembering the pain behind the hate can help us to distinguish between messages we have profound disagreements with and the messenger, a complex, multi-dimensional being, who despite their messages, has exactly the same needs as us.

I do not hope that anything I've shared in this book will help to eliminate conflict. I do not want to live in a conflict-free world! Such a world seems to me to be too sterile; too steeped in status quo; too resistant to change and supportive of mediocrity. I actually don't think polarization, division, and disagreements are the problems. They are important features of a complex, pluralistic, and democratic society. The issue is whether we react to conflict, division, and polarization with fear, avoidance, or aggression; or we develop the capacity to respond. My hope and my wish for this book is that it empowers people to respond to challenging interactions, to conflict, and to division by turning inward and then acting with clarity and strength from a place of peace and ease within.

Now, let's talk about tuning inward to solve the great issues facing the world. Actually, as Sadhguru teaches in many of his discourses, the world has but one problem—unconscious behavior by humans. You see, we are like mice in John Calhoun's mice utopia—so caught up in our own compulsions that we are not even aware of how our actions are hurling the world towards annihilation and destruction. If the problem is unconscious or compulsive behavior by humans, then the solution is moving from compulsive action to a conscious one. Conscious action means that we accept radical responsibility for the world. Radical responsibility has nothing to do with blame or causation. No, I as an American living in the southwest corner of Virginia did not cause the Taliban takeover of Afghanistan, but I am *responsible* for it. I am responsible for it because I'm not separate from the world. To illustrate this very point Sadhguru often tells a story of a philosopher fish. "A philosopher fish?" you might say while raising your eyebrows. Well, anyone could be a philosopher, why not a fish? So, a philosopher fish was swimming around asking everyone it would encounter to show it where the ocean was. The fish would share that it heard that the ocean was vast, beautiful, and mysterious and also that it had so many problems, "if only someone could help me find it," mused the philosopher fish. And, so the fish spent its entire life looking for the ocean, never realizing that not only was it *in* the ocean, it was also part of it. Radical responsibility for the world means that while I did not cause the Taliban takeover of Afghanistan nor could I do much about it, the Taliban, global warming, systemic racism, poverty, and even COVID are not separate from me; they are not happening in some alternate reality. All of these are part of me and a reflection of my consciousness. I know this is a lot to take in and to accept, but if even for a moment we consider the idea that we are not separate from the world, but that we are the world, then how we show up—whether we contribute to more peace, harmony, cohesion, or to more separation, judgment, violence matters not just for us and the people who surround us, but has much broader context and impact. Just imagine how different a place our world would be if only 10% of the seven billion people acted as though they were absolutely responsible for the world; if they committed to showing up to the extent possible for them as peace and acted with absolute awareness of the impact their actions would have on others. Wouldn't the world be a radically different place?

And, if anyone thinks an individual, a single person who commits to living from within cannot have an impact on the world, the story of Mahatma Gandhi is a great example of what is possible.

Gandhi, born Mohandas Karamchand Gandhi in Gujarat, was a shy and meager child who was an average student in school. Married at the age of thirteen in an arranged marriage to a fourteen-year-old bride, as was the custom at the time, he became a father at the age of sixteen, though Gandhi's first child died shortly after its birth. At the age of eighteen, Gandhi entered a sole, degree-granting institution in Gujarat, Samaldas College, and dropped out soon thereafter. Months later, after becoming a father to his first surviving child, Gandhi made his way to London where for the next three years he studied law at the University College of London and later at London's Inner Temple, one of the original Inns of Court, responsible for the training of barristers. Upon completion of his law studies in London, Gandhi returned to Gujarat, though was unable to make a living as a lawyer due to his shyness and inability to cross examine witnesses in court.

At the request of a client, Gandhi traveled to South Africa to handle a legal case. He ended up staying there for the next twenty-one years. It is these years in South Africa that were most formative for Gandhi. Despite being a lawyer, dressed and mannered as an English gentleman, Gandhi faced acts of intimidation and harassment due to his skin color. These acts included being thrown out from a first class rail carriage; being kicked by a police officer for walking on a white's only walking path; and being repeatedly asked by judges to remove his turban while in court. It is in response to these violent acts of discrimination that Gandhi began to formulate the enduring idea that became synonymous with his life—Satyagraha or non-violent resistance. Through various acts of satyagraha in South Africa,

Gandhi raised awareness of the plight of Indians in South Africa and unified them as a political force by founding the Natal Indian Congress. It is in South Africa that Gandhi became known as Mahatma or Great Soul.

Gandhi returned to India in 1915, at the age of forty-six to face a continent lacking in singular identity, divided by language, class, castes, ethnicity, and religions. At the time people were more likely to see themselves as Gujarati, Tamil, Telugu, Malayalam, Bengali, Punjabi, Hindu, Sikh, Jain, Christian, Muslim, or Buddhist rather than as Indian. India's people, especially in the rural areas, faced crushing poverty, limited infrastructure, inefficient bureaucracy, remnants of the centuries' old caste system, and an increasingly oppressive British mandate, which treated Indians as second-class citizens in their own land.

Upon his arrival in India, Gandhi joined the Indian National Congress and cultivated relationships with key figures, including Muslim leaders and the British Viceroy. In fact, at the request of the Viceroy, he recruited Indians to join the British Army to fight in World War I. Gandhi hoped that England would reward Indians for their loyalty with the grant of even limited swaraj, or self-rule. When that did not happen, Gandhi led the oppressed people across the country in a series of Satyagrahas—non-violent resistance campaigns. Gandhi insisted on non-violence, punctuating his insistence with hunger strikes which highlighted his willingness to die for the cause, even when the British responded with deadly force. A series of Satyagrahas which Gandhi led against the British culminated with the campaign to boycott British-made goods in India and the eventual Indian Declaration of Independence in 1930. It took England another seventeen years to recognize Indian independence. Over Gandhi's objections, whose vision was to have a unified Hindu and Muslim India, the British partitioned the sub-continent, carving out the majority-Hindu India and majority-Muslim Pakistan and Bangladesh.

A few paragraphs could hardly do justice to Gandi, the complex, multi-dimensional being that he was, and to Gandhi's nuanced and enduring legacy. Though, it is undeniable that Gandhi is a one of the fathers of modern India, whose lessons in non-violent resistance, compassion, inclusion, and loving action influenced Nelson Mandela in South Africa in his fight against Apartheid, Dr. Martin Luther King, Jr. and the U.S. Civil Rights movement, and countless others.

As Gandhi described in his autobiography, fittingly titled *The Story of My Experiments With Truth*, he was deeply influenced by the *Bhagavad Gita* and the *Upanishads*, the ancient Vedic text which focuses on the essence of living from within. Gandhi was also influenced by the writings of Leo Tolstoy, and especially Leo Tolstoy's profound philosophical treatise, *The Kingdom of God is Within You*. It is these texts that inspired Gandhi's fanatical commitment to living from within. This commitment included lifelong experiments with satya (truth), ahimsa (non-violence), santosha (simplicity or contentment), and seva (unconditional service). In fact, more than any other well known being in modern history, Gandhi embodied each of these qualities. It is embodying these qualities which enabled this shy, meager man who lived a simple, though strict monastic life to influence the world. As the man himself wrote:

> We but mirror the world. All the tendencies present in the outer world are to be found in the world of our body. If we could change ourselves, the tendencies in the world would also change. As a man changes his own nature, so does the attitude of the world change towards him. This is the divine mystery supreme. A wonderful thing it is and the source of our happiness. We need not wait to see what others do.[69]

I cannot come up with a better description and purpose of the Dis-Solving Conflict from Within process and of this book. And, to succinctly answer the questions of "so, what" and "then what," I will call on the words of the young African American poet, Amanda Gorman, who in her poem, *The Hill*

We Climb, called on a weary nation to "forge a union with purpose" and to lay down its arms "so we can reach out our arms to one another." And, finally this Sanskrit mantra, Lokah Samastah Sukhino Bhavantu, which means may all the beings be happy and free.

RESOURCES

Dis-Solving Conflict from Within™—additional recordings, guides, and daily practices www.livingpeaceinstitute.com

Mindfulness, Yoga, and Meditation:

- Anand Mehrotra and Sattva Yoga—www.sattvaconnect.com and www.mysattva.com
- Sadhguru Jaggi Vasudev—www.innerengineering.com

Conflict Resolution and Peace Building

- TRUST Network—a community of specially trained mediators and facilitators who intervene to prevent violence in protests and other volatile situations—https://mediatorsbeyondborders.org/trust/
- Braver Angels—an organization focused on bridging the political divides among Americans—https://braverangels.org/
- Mediators Beyond Borders International—an international organization, focused on promoting mediation and non-violent interventions around the world—www.mediatorsbeyondborders.com
- Center for Non-Violent Communications—offers trainings and workshops on non-violent communications https://www.cnvc.org/

- The Restorative Center—offers online and in-person Restorative Justice and Peace Circle trainings—https://www.therestorativecenter.org/
- Straus Institute of Dispute Resolution at Pepperdine Caruso Law School—one of the top graduate and professional programs in dispute resolution and peace building—https://law.pepperdine.edu/straus/
- Center for Understanding in Conflict, established by Gary Friedman, this is one of the best, integrative mediation training programs in the world—https://www.integrativelaw.com/

Conscious/Mindful/Collaborative Practice of Law

- Mindfulness in Law Society—focused on promoting mindfulness in the practice of law—https://www.mindfulnessinlawsociety.org/
- International Academy of Collaborative Professionals (IACP)—international organization, committed to promoting the practice of Collaborative Law—https://www.collaborativepractice.com/
- Integrative Law Movement—focuses on a conscious approach to the law, with special focus on Conscious Contracts—https://www.integrativelaw.com/

Further Reading:

Frankl, Viktor, *Man's Search for Meaning*
Singer, David, *Untethered Soul*
Magee, Rhonda, *The Inner Work of Racial Justice*
Rosenberg, Marshall, *Non-Violent Communications: The Language of Life*

Rippley, Amand, *High Conflict: Why We Get Trapped and How We Get Out*

Bolling, Hoffman, *Bringing Peace Into the Room*

Friedman and Himelstein, *Challenging Conflict: Mediating Through Understanding*

Cloke, Kenneth, *Mediating Dangerously*

Goldberg, Phillip, *American Veda*

Mehrotra, Anand, *This is That*

ENDNOTES

1. Dr. Sukhsimranjit Singh, Judge Danny Weinstein Managing Director and Law Professor, Straus Institute for Dispute Resolution, Pepperdine University Caruso School of Law.
2. Wallace, David Foster. "This Is Water." Kenyan College 2005 Commencement Ceremony, 2005.
3. Calhoun, John, B.; Population Density and Social Psychology, California Medicine. 113 (5): 54 (1970).
4. Id.
5. https://www.nytimes.com/interactive/2021/world/covid-cases.html, accessed on November 3, 2021.
6. Id.
7. See e.g. Aspachs O, Durante R, Graziano A, Mestres J, Reynal-Querol M, Montalvo JG (2021) Tracking the impact of COVID-19 on economic inequality at high frequency. PLoS ONE 16(3): e0249121. https://doi.org/10.1371/journal.pone.0249121.
8. IPBES (2019): Summary for policymakers of the global assessment report on biodiversity and ecosystem services of the Intergovernmental Science-Policy Platform on Biodiversity and Ecosystem Services. S. Díaz, J. Settele, E. S. Brondizio, H. T. Ngo, M. Guèze, J. Agard, A. Arneth, P. Balvanera, K. A. Brauman, S. H. M. Butchart, K. M. A. Chan, L. A. Garibaldi, K. Ichii, J. Liu, S. M. Subramanian, G.F. Midgley, P. Miloslavich, Z. Molnár, D. Obura, A. Pfaff, S. Polasky, A. Purvis, J. Razzaque, B. Reyers, R. Roy Chowdhury, Y. J. Shin, I.J. Visseren-Hamakers, K. J. Willis, and C. N. Zayas (eds.). IPBES secretariat, Bonn, Germany. 56 pages. https://doi.org/10.5281/zenodo.3553579.
9. Id.; see also https://www.nytimes.com/2019/05/06/climate/humans-are-speeding-extinction-and-altering-the-natural-world-at-an-unprecedented-pace.html?

197

10. The unclassified assessment by the U.S. Government points to two possible origins of COVID 19: human exposure to an infected animal or a lab-associated incident. See, https://www.dni.gov/files/ODNI/documents/assessments/Unclassified-Summary-of-Assessment-on-COVID-19-Origins.pdf.

11. https://www.cfr.org/backgrounder/chinas-repression-uyghurs-xinjiang.

12. https://www.bbc.com/news/world-asia-55902070.

13. https://ourworldindata.org/grapher/number-of-people-with-depression?country=~OWID_WRL.

14. See e.g. https://www.commonwealthfund.org/publications/2021/jun/building-better-systems-care-people-mental-health-problems?gclid=Cj0KCQjw5oiMBhDtARIsAJi0qk1vmFJLPpVSVRhPlbFrRyWgv7-lMN9_mkzvAWVkZEaZKHOSklPCQTMaAgIYEALw_wcB.

15. https://afsp.org/suicide-statistics/.

16. https://worldpopulationreview.com/country-rankings/suicide-rate-by-country.

17. Id.

18. Id.

19. https://jamanetwork.com/journals/jama/article-abstract/2657452.

20. https://www.drugabuse.gov/drug-topics/opioids/opioid-overdose-crisis.

21. See generally, Case, Anne, and Angus Deaton. *Deaths of Despair and the Future of Capitalism*. Princeton University Press, 2020.

22. See e.g. K.Z. Meyza, I. Ben-Ami Bartal, M.H. Monfils, J.B. Panksepp, E. Knapska, The roots of empathy: Through the lens of rodent models, *Neuroscience & Biobehavioral Reviews*, Volume 76, Part B, 2017, Pages 216–234.

23. See Genevieve Konopka, Todd F. Roberts, Animal Models of Speech and Vocal Communication Deficits Associated With Psychiatric Disorders, *Biological Psychiatry*, Volume 79, Issue 1, 2016, Pages 53–61.

24. See https://www.newscientist.com/article/dn2352-just-2-5-of-dna-turns-mice-into-men/.

25. Elisabet Sahtouris (2000) The Biology of Globalization, *World Futures*, 55:2, 105–127, DOI: 10.1080/02604027.2000.9972773.

26. Keenan, Don; Ball, David; Reptile: *The 2009 Manual of the Plaintiff's Revolution*.

27. Shapiro, Daniel; *Negotiating the Non-Negotiable: How to Resolve Your Most Emotionally Charged Conflicts*, Penguin Books (2017).

28. Names and certain identifying details were changed to protect privacy.

29. Rosen, Tommy; *Recovery 2.0: Move Beyond Addiction and Upgrade Your Life*, Hay House (2014).

30. (See, Izard, Carroll; *Human Emotions*, Springer Science & Business Media, 1977, pp. 4–17).

31. https://www.verywellmind.com/theories-of-emotion-2795717; see also, Myers, DG. Theories of Emotion, *Psychology*: Seventh Edition, Worth Publishers 2004.

32. https://explorable.com/social-judgment-theory-experiment.

33. Blythe, Will; T*o Hate Like This is To be Happy Forever: A Thoroughly Obsessive, Intermittently Uplifting, and Occasionally Unbiased Account of the Duke-North Carolina Basketball Rivalry*, HarperCollins Publishers (2007).

34. As quoted at https://billkingblog.com/what-our-founding-fathers-said-about-political-parties/.

35. Id.

36. Id.

37. See, https://news.un.org/en/story/2006/11/201222-rearing-cattle-produces-more-greenhouse-gases-driving-cars-un-report-warns; see also https://climatenexus.org/climate-issues/food/animal-agricultures-impact-on-climate-change/

38. W.F. Ritter, A.E.M. Chirnside, Impact of animal waste lagoons on ground-water quality, *Biological Wastes*, Volume 34, Issue 1, 1990, Pages 39–54.

39. Mehrotra, Anand; T*his is That: Patanjali's Yoga Sutras Padas 1 and 2*; Sattva Publications (2019), pp. 229–230.

40. Pronin, Emily; You Don't Know Me, But I Know You: The Illusion of Asymmetric Insight, *Journal of Personality and Social Psychology*, 81(4), 639–656 (2001).

41. Gladwell, Malcolm; *Talking to Strangers: What We Should Know About the People We Don't Know*, Little Brown & Company (2019).

42. www.couragetobecurious.com.

43. Rippley, Amanda; *High Conflict: Why We Get Trapped and How to Get Out*, Simon & Schuster (2021).

44. Magee, Rhonda; *The Inner Work of Racial Justice: Healing Ourselves and Transforming Our Communities Through Mindfulness*; Tarcher Perigee, New York 2019.

45. Rosenberg, Marshall; *Non-Violent Communications: The Language of Life*, PuddleDancer Press, 3rd Edition (2015).

46. Yazzie, Robert; Life Comes from It, *Navajo Justice Concepts*, 24 N.M. L. Rev. 175 (1994).

47. Id. at 179.

48. Id. at 180.

49. Brown, Howard L.; The Navajo Nation's Peacemaker's Division: An Integrated, Community-Based Dispute Resolution Forum, 24 Am. Indian L. Rev. 297 (2001).

50. Id.

51. Id.

52. Zehr, Howard; *The Little Book of Restorative Justice*, Good Books Press (2014) at p. 29.

53. Id. at p. 30.

54. Id. at appendix.

55. Pranis, Kay; *The Little Book of Circle Processes: A New/Old Approach to Peacemaking*, Good Books Press (2014).

56. Id.

57. See: https://www.therestorativecenter.org/

58. Mindfully Getting In The Middle is the title of the brilliant TEDx talk about mediation, delivered by my mentor and friend, Brad Heckman formerly of the New York Peace Institute.

59. Bush, Robert Baruch; Pope, Sally Ganong; Changing the Quality of Conflict Interaction: The Practice of Transformative Mediation, 3 Pepp. Disp. Resol. L. J. 1 (2002).

60. Cloke, Kenneth; *Mediating Dangerously: The Frontiers of Conflict Resolution*, Jossey-Bass Publishers (2001).

61. Wall, James A., Jr., Callister, Ronda Roberts; Ho'Oponopono: Some Lessons from Hawaiian Mediation, *Negotiation Journal*, January 1995, pp. 45–54.

62. Id. at p. 48, Table 1.

63. Many aspects of this model are taught by the New York Peace Institute.

64. https://www.washingtonpost.com/national/health-science/study-finds-that-fear-can-travel-quickly-through-generations-of-mice-dna/2013/12/07/94dc97f2-5e8e-11e3-bc56-c6ca94801fac_story.html.

65. See, Callaway, E. Fearful memories haunt mouse descendants. *Nature* (2013). https://doi.org/10.1038/nature.2013.14272.

66. Heisenberg, Werner (1971). Physics and Beyond: Encounters and Conversations. *World Perspectives* vol. 42. Translated by Pomerans, Arnold J. New York: Harper & Row.

67. https://blog.ted.com/qa_wih_nicholas/.

68. Baldwin, J.; *The Fire Next Time*, Vintage International (1962).

69. Gandhi, M; Vol. 13, Ch. 153, page 241, published in 1913.

ACKNOWLEDGEMENTS

The creation of this book took a village and would not be possible without many important people in my life. First and foremost, I would like to thank my wife, my life partner, Juliya Yampolsky. I dedicate this book to her as none of this would be possible without her love, patience, wisdom, her laughter and her grace. I also dedicate this book and express immense gratitude to Anand Mehrotra, my dear teacher and sweet friend. It was Anand's authentic and powerful teachings that served as the inspiration for this book. Also, I express deep gratitude to Annette Birkmann. Annette is the co-creator of the Dis-Solving Conflict from Within™ process and this book would not be possible without the immense contribution she made. My dear friend, Curtis Key, the founder of Global Collective Publishers, saw the potential in this book when so many others did not. Thank you, Curtis, for giving me a chance! Kate Stein is the brilliant editor of this book who transformed the manuscript into something suitable for human consumption. I am immensely grateful to Kate for her dedication, hard work, and attention to detail. I am grateful to my friends for their comments on the earlier versions of this manuscript. My literary agent, Christina Daigneault of Orchard Strategies provided invaluable insights about the publishing process and has also helped me improve the manuscript. Stu Webb, J. Kim Wright, David Hoffman, Woody Mosten, Pauline Tesler, Brad Heckman, Rhonda Magee, Gary Friedman, Sukhsimranjit Singh, and Kenneth Cloke are all inspirations for me in pursuing this work. I am immensely grateful to the Borland family (Kimberly, Ruth, Sarah and Joe) for their mentorship, love, and support during my family's early years in America. I am also deeply grateful to my in-laws, Rimma and Yakov Feldman and to my sister-in-law, Masha Feldman whose love, immense support, patience, and encouragement over the years has meant so much to me. When I was just a boy in Ukraine, my cousin, Leonid ("Lenchik") Braverman, first introduced me to books and ideas on communications, negotiations, and conflict which then germinated for the next thirty years. Lenchik's love, support, and humor even across continents have been deeply meaningful for me. I save the last thanks for my parents, Arnold and Rina Yampolsky. Their unconditional love made everything possible!